HOW TO HAVE
GREAT
LEGS
◆ AT ANY AGE ◆

GUYLAINE LANCTÔT, M.D.

NEW CHAPTER PRESS INC. ◆ NEW YORK

Library of Congress Catalog Card Number: 87-61130

ISBN 0-942257-04-9

Jacket design: Christopher Lione
Book design: Barbara Marks
Jacket photograph: Lynn Sugarman
Illustrations by Lynne Kopcik

To

you

and

to

my

four

children

◆ ALL MY SINCERE THANKS:

To Carola Barczak, nutrition, massage, and cellulite therapy specialist from Toronto, Canada, for your contributions to many of the chapters. All through the book, you will find information you provided me with. I appreciated your broad knowledge, your experience, and your good judgment.

To Ann Charney, writer from Montreal, Canada, for your participation in the book, and for starting this adventure with me.

To Wendy Crisp, my publisher from New York, for the concept of the book, and all the hours you have put into it. I appreciated the opportunity you gave me to work closely with you and learn from you.

To Maria Elvira dos Santos, my cook from West Palm Beach, Florida, for your precious listening and comments.

To Janine Fontaine, M.D., cardiologist and anesthesiologist from Paris, France, for all the new information and new horizons brought to medicine through your extensive research and writings about Energetic Medicine.

To Suzanne Gagnon, M.D., a dermatologist, and friend, from Montreal, Canada. Your writings about the sun and the skin have been a great help to me.

To Pamela Loftus, M.D., plastic surgeon from Boca Raton, Florida, for sharing your expertise and insight into improving the contour of our legs.

To Daisy Merey, M.D., Ph.D., bariatric physician from West Palm Beach, Florida, for providing us with the latest information on nutrition.

To Pauline Molt, fitness specialist from West Palm Beach, Florida, for your tremendous contribution to getting us in shape physically. I enjoyed greatly the many hours we spent together.

To Wayne Pickering, Sc.M., N.D., Th.D., from Daytona Beach, Florida, for sharing your knowledge and enthusiasm about nutrition and health. I was so impressed by the order in your two refrigerators—they are like your charts!

To Barbara Rien, D.P.M., podiatrist and foot surgeon from Boca Raton, Florida, for your prompt and efficient contribution of information.

To Adele Smith, professor at the Florida International University in Miami, for the latest fashion tips and your suggestions for using them with "common sense."

To Michael Vidal, L.M.T., C.T., bodywork and massage therapist from West Palm Beach, Florida. Your love and your dedication to your work impressed me as much as the gifted hands you do it with.

To Donna Zeide, M.D., dermatologist from West Palm Beach, Florida, for your enthusiastic contribution to the skin chapter.

Table Of Contents

INTRODUCTION 11

1 THE FIRST STEP 13

How Dr. Lanctôt got started with Great Legs; how you can get started with yours.

2 THE SHAPE YOU'RE IN 19

How to use the Great Legs Profile to assess the shape your legs are in now; how to plan your Great Legs Goals and your Great Legs Program.

3 THE INSIDE STORY 43

The anatomy and physiology of the leg; how five structural factors affect your legs.

4 EAT AND RUN 61

How to choose the finest fuel for your legs.

5 LIMBER LIMBS 73

How exercise affects your legs; what exercises to do for them.

6 AYE, THERE'S THE RUB 105

Massage and other techniques to make you and your legs feel great.

7 TLC — TENDER LEG CARE 115

How to have the smoothest, silkiest legs in town.

8 A GLIMPSE OF STOCKING . . . 123

What to wear to flatter and show off your Great Legs.

9 IN A SERIOUS VEIN 131

Why you get varicose veins; what you can do to prevent and treat them.

10 WALKING FOR TWO 151

How to keep your legs great during pregnancy.

11 WHY YOUR LEGS ACHE 159

. . . and what to do about it.

12 MORE THAN FAT, LESS THAN LITE 165

How you get cellulite; what you can do to get rid of it.

13 PIN-UP PERFECTION 175

Liposuction: plastic surgery for your legs.

14 LAST LEGS 181

Final encouragement for maintaining your Great Legs.

INTRODUCTION

A very simple philosophy lies at the heart of my practice of medicine. It is based on three criteria: excellence, common sense, and love. First, my work must meet the highest standards of excellence. In addition to what I have learned in my years of disciplined study and practice of medicine I demand of myself an *au courant* knowledge of scientific research, an awareness of new treatment methods, and an essential ability to interrelate all the physical and psychological systems of each human being I treat.

Second, common sense must accompany knowledge and understanding. Common sense is simply a term for judgment. In medicine, I use my judgment not only in catering to the needs of my patients but also in tending to the business aspect of my medical practice. In my clinics, my staff and I are always alert to what our patients want, because we know that meeting their requirements with excellence is the commonsense way to be successful. I believe always that I am treating a person, never a cipher. And so I use common sense in adapting and applying the principles of medicine to the needs of each person under my care.

Finally, but most important, I find it is critical not only to love my work, but also to love my patients. I care passionately about their well-being and happiness.

With love, then, I give you this book. I believe it to be filled with excellent information—accompanied, of course, by common sense!

Guylaine Lanctôt, M.D.
West Palm Beach, Florida
October 1987

THE FIRST STEP

How Dr. Lanctôt got started with Great Legs; how you can get started with yours.

◆ MY OWN KICK-OFF

My concern for legs goes back to the time shortly after I earned my M.D. I was a young physician in search of a challenge, uncertain about choosing a specialty in which to establish a practice. I knew only that I wanted to help women in a way that male physicians were, perhaps, unwilling or unable to.

At the time, I was married to a successful vascular surgeon, many of whose patients suffered from varicose veins. Although he was able, through surgery, to help patients with advanced venous disease, neither he nor his colleagues (mostly male) had much to offer the vast majority of their patients (mostly female) who had small or medium-sized varicose veins. There were few available treatments for those patients who did not need surgery but who were uncomfortable enough with their varicose veins to seek medical advice.

Historically, varicose veins have been classified as a "woman's complaint" hardly worthy of medical attention. For most doctors, treating varicose veins offers about as much glamour and prestige as attending to hemorrhoids. I was neither deterred nor intimidated by this dismissive view; on the contrary, it gave me an added incentive. I had seen the misery even small varicose veins can cause, and I decided to move in and fill this gap in medical practice.

Once my decision was made, I learned that the training I needed was not available in North America, so I left for France, where nonsurgical procedures for the treatment of varicose veins were more generally practiced. Then I returned to Canada and opened, in Montreal, my first clinic for the nonsurgical treatment of varicose veins. The response was overwhelming. Patients came from all over Canada. They told me of years of shame and humiliation, of being unable to wear shorts or go to the beach because they thought of their legs as disfigured. After treatment, they were ecstatic. Not only did they have "new and improved" legs, they also had "new and improved" feelings about their entire bodies.

It wasn't long before the number of requests for treatment demanded an expansion of the program. I opened new clinics in Montreal, Laval, and Toronto, administered by personnel I selected and trained. In 1985 I established my first U.S. clinic in Palm Beach, Florida. Since then, I have also opened clinics in Boca Raton, Miami, and Plantation, Florida.

That's all very nice Guylaine Lanctôt, you may be thinking. But what has all this to do with having Great Legs at Any Age?

In this process of treating varicose veins, I learned how dissatisfied many of us women feel about our legs and how preoccupied many of us are with our leg problems, whether real or imagined. Asked to name our best feature, very few of us nominate our legs.

In twenty years of practice, I've heard very little praise for legs, but plenty of complaints. Women tell me their legs are too fat, too skinny, too flabby, too muscular. They hate their knees, their feet, their thighs. They wish their ankles were thinner, their calves more shapely. The litany is endless. When all is said and done, however, they all want one thing: Great Legs.

This yearning is not a matter of mere vanity, I must tell you. Great Legs are critical to our health and to our general sense of well-being. What is unsightly can often be unhealthy; what is unhealthy can become unsightly. Legs reflect our overall physical and, often, psychological condition. If we're unhappy about our legs, we're likely to be unhappy with ourselves.

I say all this so that you will know that I have not written this book merely as a response to the recent rise in hemlines. Certainly, the reemergence of the miniskirt has intensified everyone's awareness of legs. But this is not a book cut to fit this year's fashions. Rather, it is a manual that tells you exactly how you can make your legs as strong, healthy, and attractive as possible. Not just this season, but every season—for the rest of your life.

Your legs are far more than objects of attention when you're wearing a short skirt or a bathing suit. They are the workhorses of your body: your primary source of mobility and locomotion. If you neglect them, your legs can become a source of pain, contributing not only to problems in walking and moving about, but also creating or aggravating back pain. As practitioners of medicine in the Far East have known for centuries, your legs are, indeed, the "roots" of your youth and vitality.

Healthy legs are attractive legs. They look young, no matter what your age. They are part of a healthy physical body. And a healthy body is one with energy that fuels accomplishment and builds self-confidence. That is why, in this book, I will give you advice on such whole-body topics as nutrition, exercise, and massage, as well as leg-specific information on such problems as varicose veins and cellulite. I have consulted many outstanding specialists, whom you will meet as I highlight their findings and programs throughout the book. In short, I'll give you all the information you need—the inside story and the outside story—to have your own Great Legs. And to keep them great at any age.

◆ YOUR PERSONAL KICK-OFF

Just as every person is unique, every person's legs are unique. So I can't present one prescription that will give every reader Great Legs. What works for one person may be counterproductive for another. You must write your own Great Legs prescription, based on your own strengths, weaknesses, and needs.

To help you determine the bare facts about your legs I have developed the Great Legs Profile, a checklist for assessing the shape you're in now. From the Profile, you will develop your Great Legs Goals. In subsequent chapters you will find the information, ideas, and exercises you will need to formulate your own Great Legs Program.

As you prepare *your* Great Legs Program, I encourage you not only to choose excellent nutrition and commonsense exercises, but also to accept, with love, the individuality of your own body.

THE SHAPE YOU'RE IN

2

How to
use the
Great Legs
Profile
to assess
the shape
your legs
are in now;
how to
plan your
Great Legs
Goals
and your
Great Legs
Program.

If you were to walk into one of my clinics the first thing I would do is sit down with you and ask you a lot of questions. Not just questions about your legs, but questions about your whole body, your lifestyle, your heredity. Remember, I treat the whole patient, not just the legs she walks in on.

I'd like you to answer these questions now yourself, as honestly and as clinically as you would if I were with you. Set aside your complaints and your negative feelings about your legs and take a good, long, objective look at them.

As you answer the questions, really look at your legs. *See* what they have to tell you. *Listen* to what your legs have to say.

You will need a quiet, private, brightly lit room with a full-length mirror. Have at hand a magnifying glass, a hand mirror, a tape measure, two scales, and a pencil to write out your answers. Also, have a pair or two of shoes available to study. Disrobe completely and stand before the mirror. Take time to think about each question before you record your answer.

◆ THE GREAT LEGS PROFILE

First, look at yourself from head to toe:
- Do you like the overall picture? Why? Why not?
- Consider the proportions of your body.
    Is there fairly good balance between your upper body and your legs?
    Do your right and left legs look significantly different from one another?
    Is one wider than the other?
    Longer?

Now, take a close look at your feet:
- Do your feet face straight forward?
- Is one foot turned out?
- Are both feet turned out?
- Are you pigeon-toed?

Step away from the mirror and examine one or two pairs of your shoes (without putting them on):

+ Do your shoes "stand up" straight?
    If not, do they incline to the inside?
    Do they spread to the outside?
+ Are the heels worn down unevenly?
+ Think about the last time you were at the beach. Did you notice your footprints in the sand?
    Were your footprints facing straight ahead?
    Did your prints show very high arches?
    Did they show flat feet?

Examine your legs for balance and straightness:

+ Are your legs the same length?
+ Are your hips level?
+ Are your knees level?
+ Are your legs straight?
    If not, are you bow-legged?
    Knock-kneed?

Turn sideways and examine your profile:

+ Is your body straight?
+ Do you tilt forward? Backward?
+ Imagine a full cup of water balanced on your head. Would the water in the cup slosh over the front of the cup? The back? Either side? (If your body is straight and your posture correct, the water should stay in the cup.)

Walk slowly toward the mirror and monitor your movement carefully:

+ Does each foot move directly forward?
+ Do your legs feel stiff?
+ Do your muscles move smoothly over one another or are they all tightened together in a mass?
+ Are you protecting a sore joint or muscle?
+ Are your movements limited?

Examine your body type:

+ Are you slim?

- Are you stocky?
- Is your body in between—slim in some places, stocky in others?
- Are you long- or short-legged?
- Do you have narrow or wide hip bones?
- Do you have narrow or wide knee bones?
- Do you have thin or thick ankle bones?

Take your dimensions. With a measuring tape, measure your thighs and calves at their fullest point.
- Are both your thighs the same size?
- Both your calves?
- Are your thighs and calves in proportion to each other? (Subtract your calf measurement from your thigh measurement. The difference should be from 6½ inches to 8½ inches.)

Weigh your "balance." Put two scales side by side and put one foot on each of them:
- Are the registered weights identical or within 15 percent of one another?
- Add both scale figures together. Are you overweight? Underweight? Check by consulting the chart below.

HEIGHT		SMALL FRAME	MEDIUM FRAME	LARGE FRAME
4 Feet	10 Inches	102-111	109-121	118-131
4	11	103-113	111-123	120-134
5	0	104-115	113-126	122-137
5	1	106-118	115-129	125-140
5	2	108-121	118-132	128-143
5	3	111-124	121-135	131-147
5	4	114-127	124-138	134-151
5	5	117-130	127-141	137-155
5	6	120-133	130-144	140-159
5	7	123-136	133-147	143-163
5	8	126-139	136-150	146-167
5	9	129-142	139-153	149-170
5	10	132-145	142-156	152-173
5	11	135-148	145-159	155-176
6	0	138-151	148-162	158-179

Source of basic data *1979 Build Study*, Society of Actuaries and Association of Life Insurance Medical Directors of America. Courtesy of the Metropolitan Life Insurance Company, 1983.

Examine your thighs:
- Are they heavy?
- Is their length and width in proportion to the rest of your body?
- Do they touch each other lightly on the inside, as they should? Is there a space between them? Are they so close together they rub uncomfortably when you walk?
- Do they have good muscle tone?
- Are the muscles tense?
- Are your thighs dimpled with fat (cellulite)?
- Do they have "saddle bags" of fat at the sides?

Examine your skin:
- Do you have enlarged veins on the insides of the thighs?
- Do you have small spider veins anywhere on the thighs?
- Do you have stretch marks?
- Does the skin sag?
- Are there blemishes or scars?
- Are you fair-skinned and sensitive to the sun?
- Are you dark-skinned and do you tan easily?

Examine your knees:
- Are they fat?
- Are they bony?
- Are they stiff or difficult to bend?
- Is the skin rough? Dry? Darker than the rest of your leg?

Examine your lower legs:
- Do you have "tube" legs (ones that don't taper)?
- Are your calves heavy?
- Do you have large muscles in your calves?
- Are there blemishes or scars?
- Is the skin dry?
- Do you have varicose veins on the inside or back of the lower leg?
- Do you have small spider veins anywhere on the lower leg?
- Are your lower legs swollen?
- Do they have good muscle tone?

◆ Can you stretch your calf muscles easily? (Test yourself by putting a thick phone book on the floor. Standing up straight and keeping your toes on the phone book, reach your heels to the floor. Can you keep this pose or is the stretch too painful?)

Look at your ankles:
◆ Do they have a fine contour?
◆ Are they lost in fat?
◆ Are they swollen?
◆ Do they have large, protruding veins?
◆ Are they weak? Do they sprain easily?
◆ Are they stiff?

Look down at your feet:
◆ Are they wide or narrow?
◆ Are they long or short?
◆ Are your feet swollen?
◆ Do you have injuries (blisters, scars) caused by shoes?
◆ Are there spider veins on your feet?
◆ Do the soles of your feet hurt when you massage them?

Stand up, close your eyes, and relax. How do your legs feel?
◆ Do they ache?
◆ Do they feel heavy?
◆ Are they tired?
◆ Are they stiff?
◆ Do they feel weak?
◆ Are they tense?
◆ Do they twitch?

Now, slip into a robe and sit comfortably to answer these final questions about your legs. Then we'll move on to questions about your lifestyle and heredity.
◆ How far can you walk without pain? One block? One mile? Five miles?
◆ Do you get leg cramps? At night?

◆ LIFESTYLE AND HEREDITY

Personal:
- ◆ Do you live in a city, a suburb, or the country?
- ◆ Is the climate warm? Cold?
- ◆ In what aspects is your personal life fulfilling?
- ◆ Do you have children?
    How many?
    Do you enjoy them?

Work:
- ◆ Do you work?
    At home?
    Outside the home?
    In an office?
- ◆ Do you work standing up?
- ◆ Do you work sitting down?
- ◆ What kind of job do you have?
    Clerical?
    Managerial?
    Manufacturing or industrial worker?
    Professional?
    Sales?
    Service?
- ◆ Is your job active?
    Sedentary?
    Creative?
    Routine?
- ◆ What is the distance between your home and your place of work?
- ◆ Do you like your job?
- ◆ Is your job extremely stressful?

Travel:
- ◆ Do you travel a lot?
    By car?
    Train?

Airplane?
Bus?
For business or pleasure?

General Health:
* Have you ever been seriously ill?
  Had surgery?
  Been badly injured?
* If so, how well did you recover?

Diet and nutrition:
* Do you eat junk food? (If you're not sure, here's a simple test. What's the difference between a Big Mac and a Whopper? If you know the answer, you eat junk food.)
* How many meals do you eat each day?
* Do you eat your meals at regular hours?
* Do you eat mostly at home or mostly in restaurants?
* How long do you spend at each meal?
* Do you enjoy cooking?
* Who does the cooking in your house?
* Can you name the basic food groups?
* Have you read a book on nutrition recently?
* Have you been on a diet? On many diets?
* Do you count calories when you eat?
* What foods do you prefer?
* Are you a meat lover?
* Are you a vegetarian?

Exercise:
* Do you exercise daily?
  Three times a week?
  Once a month?
  Never?
* Do you participate in any sports?
  In which sports do you excel?
* Do you know about or have you done aerobic exercise?
  Muscle-specific exercises?
  Stretch and tone exercises?
  Weight-resistance exercises?

- How do you spend your vacations and days off?
    At the beach?
    Skiing?
    Skating?
    Reading?
    Gardening?
    Hiking?
    Bicycling?
    Rock or mountain climbing?
    Shopping?

Heredity:
- Are your parents:
    Short and heavy?
    Tall and slim?
    Short and slight?
    Tall and heavy?
- Which parent do you most resemble physically?
- Does your mother have cellulite?
- Are your parents overweight?
- What are your parents' eating habits?
- Are there any major diseases in your family that would affect your lifestyle, diet, and exercise choices?
    Skin cancer?
    Diabetes?
    High blood pressure?
    Heart disease?
- If your parents are not living, how old were they when they died?
- Are there varicose veins on one or both sides of your family?
- Do your parents look younger or older than they are?
- Is their skin flabby and/or wrinkled?
- What kind of a child were you?
    A fat baby?
    Very active?
    Passive?
    What sports did you like?

What were your eating habits?
At what age did you begin to walk?
Did you have any major diseases as a child?

Now that you have completed your Great Legs Profile you have not only become thoroughly acquainted with your legs, but you have a good understanding of the other factors that affect the shape your legs are in—your lifestyle, diet and nutrition, exercise, and heredity. Of course, you cannot change your heredity, but you can change your lifestyle and give up poor diet and exercise habits that adversely affect the shape of your legs.

Throughout the book you'll find advice that addresses your specific problems and weaknesses. For example, if you live in a cold climate with severe winters, you could well have a problem with dry skin. You'll want to pay special attention to the section on keeping skin smooth in Chapter 7. If you have an unusually stressful job, you may want to try one of the massage methods described in Chapter 6 for its relaxing effects as well as its benefits to your legs.

◆ YOUR GREAT LEGS GOALS—THE SHAPE YOU WILL BE IN

What are Great Legs? Great Legs are first and foremost healthy legs. They are strong, straight, in proportion to the rest of your body, well-toned, limber, and free of excess fat. They are not swollen or discolored. Their skin is smooth and supple.

But what are *your* Great Legs? They are the best legs *you* can have. They are unlike anyone else's Great Legs. They are yours and yours alone. Only you can make them.

There is room below for you to set five goals for your Great Legs. (By all means set more—or less—if that suits you.) Work from your Great Legs Profile, remembering to keep your goals specific and attainable. If you come from a family of women with wide hips and short legs, you will never have narrow hips and long legs, but you *can* learn to dress in a way that will make your hips seem narrower and your legs seem longer.

Setting a realistic time frame for achieving each of your Great Legs Goals will give you the impetus to keep working and a concrete way to monitor your progress.

MY GREAT LEGS GOALS

1.

2.

3.

4.

5.

◆ YOUR GREAT LEGS PROGRAM

Now that you have chosen excellent goals, the next step is setting up a commonsense program for achieving them. The information in this book will enable you to do just that. As you read, note the information that addresses your specific goals. Plan your strategy and write your program in the space provided below.

Good luck! I am certain you are going to love your Great Legs.

MY GREAT LEGS PROGRAM

Goal 1

Goal 2

Goal 3

Goal 4

Goal 5

To show you how easy it is to create your own Great Legs Program I asked Marie Fiore to share hers with you. Marie lives in Yonkers, New York, and works as a computer consultant for a large food manufacturing company in nearby White Plains, New York. Her husband, Jack, is a lawyer, and they have two sons, aged seven and ten. Marie is thirty-eight and grew up in Brooklyn, New York.

◆ SAMPLE GREAT LEGS PROFILE, GOALS AND PROGRAM

First, look at yourself from head to toe:

• Do you like the overall picture? Why? Why not?
Not bad for thirty-eight and a working mother of two. A few extra pounds and inches here and there and my legs are starting to get veins like Mom's, but overall, not bad at all.

• Consider the proportions of your body.
Is there fairly good balance between your upper body and your legs? Yes.
Do your right and left legs look significantly different from one another? Is one wider than the other? Longer? No, they look about equal to me.

Now, take a close look at your feet:

• Do your feet face straight forward? No.
• Is one foot turned out? No.
• Are both feet turned out? Yes, slightly.
• Are you pigeon-toed? No.

Step away from the mirror and examine one or two pairs of your shoes (without putting them on):

• Do your shoes "stand up" straight? No.
If not, do they incline to the inside? Yes, slightly.
Do they spread to the outside? No.
• Are the heels worn down unevenly? Yes, more on the inside.
• Think about the last time you were at the beach. Did you notice your footprints in the sand? I think I remember them.
Were your footprints facing straight ahead? No, toes turn out.
Did your prints show very high arches? No.
Did they show flat feet? No, but very low arches.

Examine your legs for balance and straightness:
- Are your legs the same length? Yes.
- Are your hips level? Yes.
- Are your knees level? Yes.
- Are your legs straight? Yes.
    If not, are you bow-legged? No.
    Knock-kneed? No.

Turn sideways and examine your profile:
- Is your body straight? Yes.
- Do you tilt forward? A little bit. Backward? No.
- Imagine a full cup of water balanced on your head. Would the water in the cup slosh over the front of the cup? The back? Either side? (If your body is straight and your posture correct, the water should stay in the cup.) Looks pretty straight to me. I guess all those dancing lessons as a kid paid off.

Walk slowly toward the mirror and monitor your movement carefully:
- Does each foot move directly forward? No, toes turn out.
- Do your legs feel stiff? A little.
- Do your muscles move smoothly over one another or are they all tightened together in a mass? Move smoothly.
- Are you protecting a sore joint or muscle? No.
- Are your movements limited? No.

Examine your body type:
- Are you slim? Yes, except thighs.
- Are you stocky? No.
- Is your body in between—slim in some places, stocky in others? Okay, except thighs.
- Are you long- or short-legged? Long.
- Do you have narrow or wide hip bones? Narrow.
- Do you have narrow or wide knee bones? Narrow.
- Do you have thin or thick ankle bones? Thin.

Take your dimensions. With a measuring tape, measure your thighs and calves at their fullest point.

♦ Are both your thighs the same size? Right,23"; Left,23"
♦ Both your calves? Right,14"; Left,14"
♦ Are your thighs and calves in proportion to each other? (Subtract your calf measurement from your thigh measurement. The difference should be from 6-1/2 inches to 8-1/2 inches.) 9" difference—thighs need work.

Weigh your "balance." Put two scales side by side and put one foot on each of them:

♦ Are the registered weights identical or within 15 percent of one another? Yes.
♦ Add both scale figures together. 124 pounds.
  Are you overweight? Underweight? According to the chart, I'm okay.

Examine your thighs:

♦ Are they heavy? Yes.
♦ Is their length and width in proportion to the rest of your body? Seem wide in relation to the rest of my body, which is generally narrow.
♦ Do they touch each other lightly on the inside, as they should? Is there a space between them? Are they so close together they rub uncomfortably when you walk? They rub a little. Not exactly uncomfortable, but I'm aware of it.
♦ Do they have good muscle tone? No, flabby!
♦ Are the muscles tense? A little.
♦ Are your thighs dimpled with fat (cellulite)? Some ripples in the back and on the sides.
♦ Do they have "saddle bags" of fat at the sides? Bulge at each side, yes.
♦ How does the skin look? Dry, flaky.
♦ Do you have enlarged veins on the insides of the thighs? No.
♦ Do you have small spider veins anywhere on the thighs? Yes, some.
♦ Do you have stretch marks? Not on thighs, only on tummy.

- Does the skin sag? Not yet. (Let's keep it that way.)
- Are there blemishes or scars? No.
- Are you fair-skinned and sensitive to the sun? No.
- Are you dark-skinned and do you tan easily? Yes.

Examine your knees:
- Are they fat? No.
- Are they bony? Not especially.
- Are they stiff or difficult to bend? No.
- Is the skin rough? Dry? Darker than the rest of your leg? Rough and dry but not darker.

Examine your lower legs:
- Do you have "tube" legs (ones that don't taper)? No.
- Are your calves heavy? No.
- Do you have large muscles in your calves? No.
- Are there blemishes or scars? No.
- Is the skin dry? Yes.
- Do you have varicose veins on the inside or back of the lower leg? No.
- Do you have small spider veins anywhere on the lower leg? Some.
- Are your lower legs swollen? No.
- Do they have good muscle tone? Not bad; better than my thighs.
- Can you stretch your calf muscles easily? (Test yourself by putting a thick phone book on the floor. Standing up straight and keeping your toes on the phone book, reach your heels to the floor. Can you keep this pose or is the stretch too painful?) Not painful, but I feel the stretch.

Look at your ankles:
- Do they have a fine contour? Yes, if I do say so myself.
- Are they lost in fat? No.
- Are they swollen? No.
- Do they have large, protruding veins? No.
- Are they weak? Do they sprain easily? No.
- Are they stiff? No.

Look down at your feet:
- ◆ Are they wide or narrow? No. Average in length and width.
- ◆ Are they long or short? Average.
- ◆ Are your feet swollen? No.
- ◆ Do you have injuries (blisters, scars) caused by shoes? Yes, "pump bumps."
- ◆ Are there spider veins on your feet? No.
- ◆ Do the soles of your feet hurt when you massage them? One tender spot.

Standing up, close your eyes, and relax. How do your legs feel?
- ◆ Do they ache? No.
- ◆ Do they feel heavy? No.
- ◆ Are they tired? Could have more pep.
- ◆ Are they stiff? A little.
- ◆ Do they feel weak? No.
- ◆ Are they tense? A little.
- ◆ Do they twitch? No.

Now, slip into a robe and sit comfortably to anwer these final questions about your legs. Then we'll move on to questions about your lifestyle and heredity.
- ◆ How far can you walk without pain? One block? One mile? Five miles? Two or three miles.
- ◆ Do you get leg cramps? No. At night? No.

◆ LIFESTYLE AND HEREDITY

Personal:
- ◆ Do you live in a city, a suburb, or the country? Suburb.
- ◆ Is the climate warm? Cold? Cold.
- ◆ In what aspects is your personal life fulfilling? Jack and I have a really good, supportive marriage. I could do with some more time for myself, but with a job, a home and two kids...

◆ Do you have children? Yes.

    How many? Two.

    Do you enjoy them? They're great!

Work:

◆ Do you work? Yes.

    At home? If you count housework—which I do!

    Outside the home? Yes.

    In an office? Yes.

◆ Do you work standing up? Sometimes.

◆ Do you work sitting down? Mostly.

◆ What kind of job do you have?

    Clerical?

    Managerial?

    Manufacturing or industrial worker?

    Professional? Yes.

    Sales?

    Service?

◆ Is your job active? Somewhat—lots of running between departments and work stations.

    Sedentary? Can be, when I'm designing a new system or have a lot of paperwork to catch up on.

    Creative? I sure have to be on my toes.

    Routine? No way, there's always some fire to fight.

◆ What is the distance between your home and your place of work? Ten miles.

◆ Do you like your job? Most of the time.

◆ Is your job extremely stressful? It can be.

Travel:

◆ Do you travel a lot? Not as much as I'd like to, for pleasure, that is.

    By car? Drive to work—fifteen minutes each way.

    Train? Rarely.

    Airplane? Occasionally.

    Bus? Rarely.

    For business or pleasure? Both.

General Health:

♦ Have you ever been seriously ill? No.
   Had surgery? Tonsils removed as a child.
   Been badly injured? No.
♦ If so, how well did you recover? Pretty well, as far as I remember.

Diet and nutrition:

♦ Do you eat junk food? (If you're not sure, here's a simple test. What's the difference between a Big Mac and a Whopper? If you know the answer, you eat junk food.) Guess I don't eat junk food, although I don't mind a chocolate ice cream cone now and then.
♦ How many meals do you eat each day? Three.
♦ Do you eat your meals at regular hours? Usually.
♦ Do you eat mostly at home or mostly in restaurants? Home.
♦ How long do you spend at each meal? Breakfast—twenty minutes; dinner—forty-five minutes; lunch is catch as catch can.
♦ Do you enjoy cooking? Yes.
♦ Who does the cooking in your house? Cook mostly on weekends and freeze weekday meals. Jack and boys help.
♦ Can you name the basic food groups? Sure—grains, fruits and vegetables, dairy, meats.
♦ Have you read a book on nutrition recently? Magazine and newspaper articles only.
♦ Have you been on a diet? On many diets? Only after kids were born.
♦ Do you count calories when you eat? No.
♦ What foods do you prefer? Pasta, fresh fruits and vegetables, the odd slice of pizza.
♦ Are you a meat lover? No.
♦ Are you a vegetarian? No, but we eat very little meat.

Exercise:

♦ Do you exercise daily? Wish I had time!
   Three times a week? I try.

Once a month? More than that—about twice a week generally.

Never?

+ Do you participate in any sports? Cross-country skiing, bicycling.

In which sports do you excel? Can't say I'm a great sportswoman, but I enjoy being active.

+ Do you know about or have you done aerobic exercise? Yes, aerobic classes at health club.

Muscle-specific exercises? Yes.

Stretch and tone exercises? Yes.

Weight-resistance exercises? Use machines at health club sometimes.

+ How do you spend your vacations and days off?

At the beach? Sometimes.

Skiing? Whenever possible.

Skating? No.

Reading? Frequently.

Gardening? Frequently.

Hiking? Whenever possible.

Bicycling? Whenever possible.

Rock or mountain climbing? Not with my head for heights!

Shopping? Only if absolutely necessary.

Heredity:

+ Are your parents:

Short and heavy? No.

Tall and slim? Mom—average height and slim.

Short and slight? Dad's on the short side, slight except for pot belly.

Tall and heavy?

+ Which parent do you most resemble physically? Mom.

+ Does your mother have cellulite? No.

+ Are your parents overweight? Dad's a little overweight now that he's older; was not as a young man.

+ What are your parents' eating habits? Mom sticks to meals, Dad's a snacker, especially fruit and "nibbles." Neither has a sweet tooth.

39

- Are there any major diseases in your family that would affect your lifestyle, diet, and exercise choices?

    Skin cancer? No.

    Diabetes? No.

    High blood pressure? No.

    Heart disease? No.

- If your parents are not living, how old were they when they died? Both still living.

- Are there varicose veins on one or both sides of your family? Mom's side.

- Do your parents look younger or older than they are? Younger, about ten years.

- Is their skin flabby and/or wrinkled? No.

- What kind of child were you?

    A fat baby? No.

    Very active? Yes.

    Passive? No.

    What sports did you like? Bicycling, swimming.

    What were your eating habits? Like parents—healthy meals, few sweets, soda only on special occasions.

    At what age did you begin to walk? Mom said eleven months.

    Did you have any major diseases as a child? No.

MARIE'S GREAT LEGS GOALS

1. Thinner, firmer thighs.

2. More exercise. Could be why I've been feeling tired and stiff lately.

3. Find out why my feet are everted and hips distorted. Could be the cause of back pain???

4. Hadn't looked at my veins for a while. A few more varicose veins than I had thought. Learn about prevention and treatment, especially since Mom has them.

5. Moist, supple skin on legs.

MARIE'S GREAT LEGS PROGRAM

Goal 1

1. Do muscle-specific workout, Chapter 5, three times per week. Fit in after work while watching evening news.

2. Follow fashion suggestions, Chapter 8, to camouflage thighs until I can get them in shape.

Goal 2

Switch from bike riding to fitness walking, thirty minutes three times per week. Make the effort to get up forty-five minutes earlier in the morning to do this. Make sure to stretch before and after working out. This should help my energy level and that stiffness I've been feeling lately.

Goal 3

Call Dr. Adams for referral to orthopedic surgeon. Make appointment to see about my hip and leg distortion. Chapter 3 has proved to me how important this is. My whole spine may be out of whack because of this distortion and it is more than likely causing my backaches. Fix this now so I don't develop any more problems.

If not a medical problem, see a massage or body work therapist.

Goal 4

Keep exercising and invest in some attractive support hose to prevent more varicose veins, as prescribed in Chapter 11. See a vein specialist to discuss current status of my veins and treatment options.

Goal 5

For smoother, moist skin, use loofah before bathing. Watch water temperature—usually make my baths too hot. (Not good for veins either.) Remember to blot dry with towel, not rub after bath or shower.

Goal 6

Make more time for a nutritious and relaxed lunch.

The Inside Story

The anatomy and physiology of the leg; how five structural factors affect your legs.

G reat Legs are strong, healthy, and attractive. But what makes them that way? To find out, we need to take a closer look at the physical structure of our legs and learn something about how they work. We also need to examine the five factors that influence the physical state of our legs: heredity, balance, feet, gait, and posture.

◆ THE PHYSICAL STRUCTURE OF THE LEG

Medically speaking, your legs constitute the part of your lower limbs between your knees and your ankles. Above your knees are your thighs—officially not considered part of your legs. (Considering how some women feel about their thighs, this should come as great news!) Your thighs extend from your knees to your hips. Your derrière is excluded from this territory. Departing from medical practice, I will refer to the entire lower limb—from groin to ankle—as your leg.

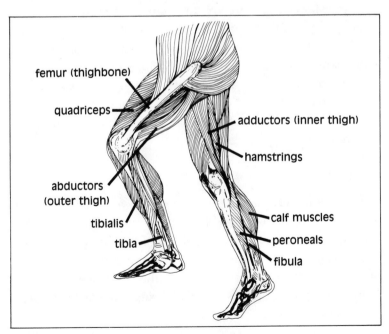

45

BONES

The bone in your thigh is called the femur. In the lower leg, there are two bones: the tibia (the shin bone) and the fibula (the long, thin, outer bone).

MUSCLES

Your thigh muscles can be divided into four groups:
* the quadriceps (quads), in front of the thigh. They are likely to ache after strenuous walking, bicycling, climbing, or lifting heavy objects.
* the hamstrings, in the back of the thigh. If you bend over, keeping your knees straight, you will feel the pull on your hamstrings.
* the abductors, in the outer thigh. They move your leg away from the body.
* the adductors, in the inner thigh. They move your leg toward the body.

In your lower leg, there are three groups of muscles:
* the tibialis, in the front of the leg. They flex your foot at the ankle. (Paralysis of the tibialis anterior causes foot drop.)
* the calf muscles, which form the bulge of the calf that is noticeable in athletes' and dancers' calves. They extend your foot at the ankle.
* the peroneals, at the outer side of your leg, which support the arch of the foot.

NERVES

The sciatic nerve is the largest nerve in your body and also the main nerve in your legs. Branches of nerves in your lower back meet at each side of your pelvis to form the sciatic nerve. The sciatic extends from your pelvis down through your derrière, then behind your hip joint to the back of your thigh. Above the knee, it divides in two and runs along both the peroneal muscles and the tibia bone.

The other important leg nerve is the femoral nerve. Coming

in from your groin, the femoral nerve extends down through your leg, closely following the path of the femoral artery.

ARTERIES AND VEINS

The heart pumps oxygenated blood to the leg mainly through the femoral artery. Provided you don't have arteriosclerosis (hardening of the arteries), arterial blood has a comparatively easy time reaching your legs. The heart pumps continuously, and gravity works in its favor.

Venous blood, on the other hand, does not have an easy time of it in your legs. The job of your veins is to return oxygen-depleted blood to the heart, so it can be reoxygenated in the lungs and redistributed throughout the body by the arteries. The blood must flow uphill in the veins. Unlike the arteries, they have no central pumping station (that is, the heart) to assist them in this task. Gravity, obviously, is an obstacle.

So, what pumps the blood up from your feet to your heart? It is done by the muscular "pump" in each of your legs, particularly the calf muscles and the peroneal muscles. As you walk, these muscles contract, squeezing the deep veins in your legs and forcing the blood upward.

At intervals along the insides of the veins there are simple valves. When these valves work properly, they ensure that the blood can move in one direction only: back to your heart. When these valves don't work properly, blood will collect in your veins like backwater in a swamp. If the muscles in your legs are weak from lack of exercise or from atrophy following an illness, the pumping system will not work as it should.

There are two main vein systems—the deep and the superficial.

The **deep vein system,** located deep inside your legs, carries 90 percent of the blood that is returned to your heart. The deep veins lie beneath muscles, which surround and contain them. The muscles prevent the deep veins from becoming dilated, or expanded. When deep veins are damaged, they can cause major problems, such as those in the postphlebitic syndrome. In this condition blood flows the wrong way in the veins.

It is marked by pain, swelling, and discoloration of the leg. Physicians have no direct access to deep veins but diagnosis of deep vein illness can be made through instruments such as X ray or ultrasound.

The **superficial vein system**, which carries 10 percent of the blood that returns to your heart, is located just beneath the skin. Unlike the deep vein system, it can be seen and felt; physicians can diagnose its conditions by sight and touch. While deep veins are surrounded by strong muscle, only the skin keeps superficial veins from dilating and becoming varicose. (A varicose vein is one that is dilated and nonfunctioning—known as "incompetent" in medical parlance.)

When blood does not flow properly through a vein but instead stagnates, the skin tissue surrounding the vein cannot receive the nutrition the blood carries. The nutrition of the skin becomes impaired.

Among the superficial veins that can become varicose, the saphenous veins are the most important for two reasons: they are the largest of the superficial veins, and they are often affected by heredity.

I will discuss the prevention and treatment of varicose veins later; but for now, it is important to recognize the crucial relationship between your muscles and your veins.

THE LYMPHATIC SYSTEM

Like the vein system, the lymphatic system also relies on the muscles to pump tissue fluid, called lymph, along its vessels. Also like veins, these vessels converge—smaller ones to larger ones—and eventually empty the lymph into the two largest veins near the heart.

Lymph, a warm, saline solution, is the part of the blood that delivers the nutrients each cell needs to stay alive. Once tissues have derived nutrients from the lymph, the used fluid must drain away through the lymph vessels. If it didn't, the body would blow up like a balloon. Poor lymph drainage is often the cause of swollen legs.

The lymphatic system also has lymph nodes where the body manufactures disease-fighting lymphocytes. Invading organisms are carried in the lymph to the nodes, where the lymphocytes work to neutralize them. So good lymph drainage is also important for maintaining good health.

THE ENERGETIC AND SPIRITUAL BODIES

Many Western-trained physicians would stop a discussion of anatomy and physiology here. Because of their training (the same that I received) they consider only the physical body when diagnosing and curing patients. They take into account only what they can observe, touch, and analyze. By paying attention to the material, physical body, modern Western medicine has made tremendous strides in curing diseases and improving longevity. No one can or should dispute that.

In the course of my studies in France, however, I learned that there are other theories about the body, theories based on ancient beliefs and Eastern medical practices. Recently, these theories have been gaining currency in the West. One such theory suggests that the human being has, in addition to a physical body, bodies of energy and spirit as well. In my quest for more knowledge about energy, I met in Paris with Dr. Janine Fontaine. Dr. Fontaine is a physician, cardiologist, and anesthesiologist who has devoted her practice and her writings over the last eighteen years to Energetic Medicine.

The **energetic body** cannot be seen or measured, and so it is a difficult concept to grasp. It derives from energy that circulates inside our physical body along invisible pathways called meridians. (These are the pathways used in acupuncture and Shiatsu, or acupressure massage.) Outside the physical body, the energetic body vibrates in invisible circular layers that are something like the circle of ripples in a pond when a stone is thrown into it. It has its own rules. Any alteration in the normal structure of the energetic body can lead to illness.

As I've said before, our legs play a very big part in our overall physical and mental health. Greater awareness of the flow of energy in and around the physical body—and awareness of those times when the energetic body is impeded or blocked—can improve not only physical but mental well-being.

Like our energetic body, the **spiritual body** is made up of vibrations and it never dies. This nonmaterial entity—an intimate part of ourselves—connects with the universe independently of time and space. We can only understand the concept of the spiritual body with our intuition and our perception. Our intellect cannot teach us anything about the spirit because the intellect is strictly oriented toward material substance.

The status of the spiritual body has a great effect on our health. Improving its condition improves our health.

When thinking about and planning for your Great Legs, please remember the power of *your* energy and spirit.

◆ FIVE FACTORS THAT INFLUENCE THE STATE OF YOUR LEGS

Clothes, no matter how fashionable, will only look as great as the body that wears them. A body can only look as great as its underlying structure allows. The same, of course, goes for your legs.

The underlying structure of your legs is determined by five factors: heredity, balance, feet, gait, and posture. Let's take a closer look at each of these.

HEREDITY

For the most part, the look of your legs has been determined by your ancestors; diet and exercise have lesser roles. Your genes dictate general shape: the length of your bones, the width of your tendons, and the proportion of fast- and slow-twitch fibers in your leg muscles.

Muscle Fibers

If you've inherited mostly slow-twitch muscle fibers, you have thin legs that may be lacking in roundness, shape, and definition. Slow-twitch muscle fibers are long and thin and are found in small-boned people who have small joints and narrow tendons. You see slow-twitch legs on marathon runners, ballet dancers, and long-distance walkers.

If your legs are broad, with a wide Achilles tendon and thick, rounded heels, you have mostly fast-twitch muscle fibers. You're probably big-boned and wide-jointed as well. Fast-twitch legs are powerful and good for sprinting. You see them in track and field athletes and tennis players.

You can't change your basic muscle fiber type, nor should you want to. A majority of slow-twitch muscle fibers simply wouldn't suit a big-boned, wide-jointed person. Through exercise, and to some extent diet, you can modify the ratio of fast- to slow-twitch fibers. Here's what you can do.

For thinner legs with a longer, leaner look and fewer fast-twitch fibers:

+ Choose walking, running, or swimming for cardiovascular fitness.
+ Never exercise your legs for less than thirty minutes.
+ Never use leg weights.
+ Avoid excessive intake of protein.

For shapelier legs with more contours and fewer slow-twitch fibers:

+ Take up weight-resistance training.
+ Choose racket sports, bicycling, or rowing for cardiovascular fitness.
+ Use ankle weights.
+ Increase the amount of protein in your diet.

Hips

Wide hips are an inherited body type that cannot be changed. You cannot diet or exercise your way to narrow hips. Nor can you have "fat," which is not the villain here, surgically removed.

You can:

+ Always keep your weight within the normal to low-normal range; extra weight exaggerates hip width.
+ Exercise for maximum trimness and muscle tone.

Knees

With skirt hems flirting with thighs these days, our knees—for better or worse—are attracting attention. This is not great news for these of you who identified a wide knee bone (patella) on your Great Legs Profile. A wide patella makes your knees appear "fat," even when they are not. As with wide hips, surgery can do nothing to improve the appearance of your knees.

You can:

◆ Avoid leg exercises that will build up the muscle around your knees.

◆ Lower your hemlines to a half-inch below the knee.

You will have to live with whatever heredity has decided for you. You may be able to change and improve some things, but others will remain the same, no matter what you do.

This will be easier to accept if you learn to love your body. If you were born short, convince yourself that small people are the greatest. If you feel you are too tall, think of all the reasons it is wonderful to be tall. You cannot overcome your heredity, but you can make a lasting peace with it.

BALANCE

Balanced legs are a sign of a balanced body. The body is a well-organized structure in which all the parts are interrelated. When one part goes askew, it causes all the others to go askew. For instance, everted (turned out) feet induce everted ankles, knees, and hips. Everted feet can also cause a distortion in the spine and many secondary problems.

Balanced legs are even in:

◆ Length
◆ Weight
◆ Muscular strength
◆ Orientation

You tested for right-left imbalance in the Great Legs Profile by observing yourself in the mirror and when you stood on two scales. If you noticed an imbalance, the next pages will be of special interest to you.

Uneven Legs

By comparing the height of the front bone tips of your hip bones, you will know immediately if your legs are uneven. If your hip bones are level, good for you. If they are not, your shoulders will also look uneven.

If you find you have an imbalance, you should consult your physician or an orthopedic surgeon as soon as possible. The doctor will examine you for any bone malformation or disease. If those are ruled out, he or she will determine the cause of your imbalance. Once the original problem is identified and corrected (either by treatment or by an orthopedic device worn in your shoe), the rest of your body will get back to normal.

In any case, uneven legs are a condition that should be treated. Left alone, the imbalance can cause many problems, such as chronic muscular pain, joint pain, or back pain.

Distortion of the Pelvis

A distorted, or rotated, pelvis is one in which the hip joint is not in its normal position. Normally, the pelvis relates the hip

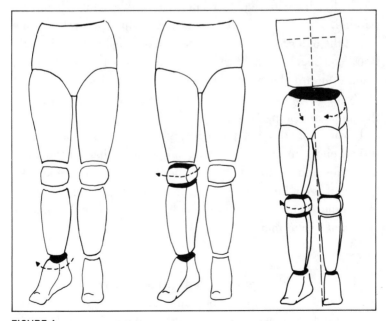

FIGURE 1

joint to the femoral bone in a way that ensures smooth working of the joint.

Look at the figures in Figure 1. From left to right they show how a turned-out foot is a sign of pelvic rotation. The foot is turned out and the knee is distorted because of the pelvis distortion on both the horizontal and vertical axes. Although not shown in this diagram, the spine, too, is distorted.

Pelvic rotation has many causes. It may begin early in life with too-heavy diapering, for instance, which requires the child to walk spread-legged around the thick barrier of cloth. Walking too soon can also cause pelvic rotation. Or it can be caused by accident or disease.

If you have such a distortion, it should be examined and treated by a physician or orthopedic surgeon as soon as possible. Like imbalance of the legs, untreated pelvic rotation can also cause secondary problems like muscular, joint, and back pain.

Knee and Ankle Rotations

Ideally, the movement of knee and ankle joints should be parallel. That is, the joints themselves should be centered one above the other to ensure movement in a straight forward direction. You checked this during your Great Legs Profile when you walked toward the mirror. If your feet pointed straight ahead and your knees were parallel to your ankles as you walked, then the joints are properly aligned.

If your feet did not point straight ahead and your knees turned either in or out, you have a condition that warrants examination and treatment. If your knees turn out, you are knock-kneed; if your knees turn in, you are bowlegged. Both these aberrations can cause such secondary problems as leg imbalance and pelvic rotation.

FEET

The foot's vital function is to distribute adequately the pressure of standing, walking, and running. A three-part arch system in the foot transmits and distributes the weight of the body

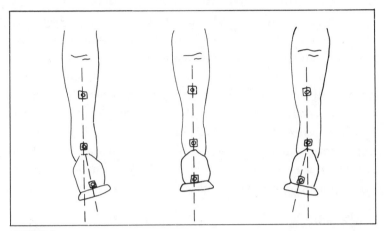

FIGURE 2

during any activity. The arch of the foot is determined by the alignment of the knee and ankle, along with the integrity of the muscles of the lower leg.

Let's take a look at the foot from the back. In Figure 2, you see three different alignments of the foot and leg: pronation, the neutral position, and supination. In a pronation position, the line from mid-calf to the center of the heel turns out, causing the weight to be borne on the inside of the foot. In the neutral position, the line from mid-calf to the center of the heel is straight; the weight is correctly distributed. In the supination position, the line from mid-calf to the center of the heel turns in, causing the weight to be borne on the outside of the foot.

If you look at the foot from the front, you will see that in the pronation position the toes are turned out (everted). In the neutral position the toes are pointed straight ahead, as they should be. In the supination position, the toes are turned in (inverted).

Flat Feet

Feet are flat because the bones of the foot are not held up in an arch. The peroneal muscles of the lower leg literally hoist up the arch. When, for whatever reason, they do not do that job, the feet are flat.

Many patients tell me they were "born" with flat feet, that flat feet run in their families. The problem, however, is not only heredity but the state of the muscles when the child begins to walk. If the muscles are not strong enough to interact properly with one another, the arch will not form.

You may have been "born" with flat feet, but you need not die with them. Your muscles can be repatterned to work together correctly through physical therapy. Some of the massage and body work systems described in Chapter 6 include techniques for reeducating underused or poorly used muscles. Your physician or a podiatrist may be able to recommend an appropriate practitioner in your area.

Tracks

In the Great Legs Profile I asked you to remember or look at your footprints at the beach. These are your tracks. You can get a great deal of information about your body alignment from them.

Look at Figure 3. What kind of tracks would this car make?

Wheels that track like those in the illustration cannot roll with any real speed because they are not moving straight ahead in tandem. Also, every turn of an unbalanced wheel erodes its axle and limits the useful life of the whole system.

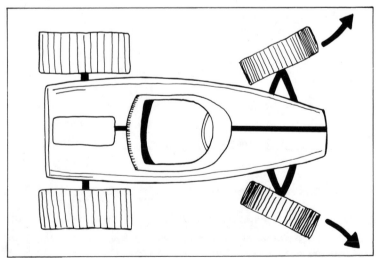

FIGURE 3

Much the same is true of feet. Turned-out tracks like the ones in Figure 4 are the result of turned-out feet. Chronic eversion of the feet causes the peroneal muscles (the ones that hoist the arch) to become chronically shortened. The muscles do not move smoothly and in concert with each other. Instead, they work as if they were practically glued together. This not only impedes speed and balance, but misaligns the whole body as well.

I think you can see now why it is so very important to have balanced legs and straight-facing feet. If you have noticed an imbalance in your legs or a pronation or supination of your feet, consult a physician to have the condition examined and corrected. Your Great Legs depend on it.

GAIT

How many times have you seen someone from the back or at a distance too great to distinguish her face? "That must be Helen," you say. "I'd know her walk anywhere."

Your gait is not only distinctive but also gives a lot of clues to your body alignment. The ideal gait starts with feet that face straight forward. Straight-facing feet allow the ankles and knees to move as they are meant to move—in a forward-and-back-

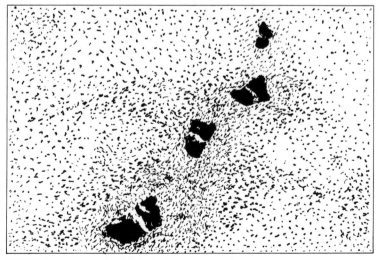

FIGURE 4

ward motion much like that of a door hinge. If the feet do not face forward and the ankle and knee "hinges" do not work properly, the result could be a pelvic rotation—or some other misalignment.

Unfortunately, most people have a toed-out gait, as you will see if you examine footprints the next time you are at the beach. If your toes face any way but straight ahead as you walk, it would be well worth your while to have yourself examined for leg imbalance or joint rotation and to take measures to correct that imbalance. Then you can work on reeducating your muscles. A strong, balanced gait can only enhance your Great Legs.

POSTURE

I'm sure your mother, like mine, told you to stand up straight more times than she or you would like to remember. Unfortunately, many of us have forgotten our mothers' good advice. Or we have developed problems—flat feet, for instance—that have affected our posture.

Look at the two profiled figures in Figure 5. In Profile A the weight droops downward, as if it is in a losing battle with gravity. Posture like this can lead to many problems: hyper-extended legs, distorted pelvis, exaggerated spinal curve, sagging rib cage, or dowager's hump (a fat pad that has grown to protect the sore juncture of the upper spine with the neck).

In Profile B, however, the body seems to lift, not droop. It seems to have an imaginary "skyhook" pulling it up. Notice how the horizontal and vertical lines bisecting Profile B meet at right angles. The horizontal lines do not slope downward, as in Profile A.

Acquiring posture like the one in Profile B is crucial to your Great Legs. Why? Because, as I have said before, all the structures in the body are interrelated. If your posture is lax and sagging, how can your legs be firm and straight?

Remember when standing tall that your knees should always be loose (slightly bent, not locked), so that your body weight is supported by the quadriceps (thigh) muscles instead of your lower back. When you contract your abdominal muscles and tuck your derrière under slightly, the lower back is adequately supported. Shoulders should be relaxed and open, not drawn up toward your ears, hunched over, or excessively pulled back. Remember also to keep your neck straight; your chin should neither droop down nor point up.

Correct posture will improve your appearance, relieve lower back stress, and put your thigh muscles to work for more attractive legs. It is also good for your psychological health. The way you stand says a lot about you. It is a hallmark of the image you present to the world. Don't forget that the image you project to others comes back to you, which in turn influences your self-image profoundly.

So, remember to stand up tall on your Great Legs and meet the world proudly and confidently.

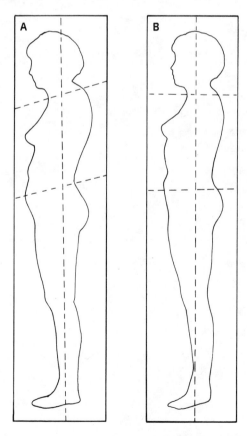

FIGURE 5

Eat And Run

How to choose the finest fuel for your legs.

The food you eat is to your body what gasoline is to your car. If you don't have gas, the car won't go; if you use bad gas, you will damage the car. When you don't eat well, your body does not run properly. And if your body is functioning at less than its optimum level, your legs will not be as strong and healthy as they can be. You can only have healthy legs with good nutrition.

Eating is one thing; eating *well* is quite another. What does it mean to eat well? It means providing your body with the best ingredients, in sensible portions, at the times your body needs fuel. Eating well also means eating in a relaxed, pleasant atmosphere. Mealtime is not the time for arguments—or for television. You need to have positive thoughts while you eat so your food will be converted into positive energy.

Eating is, on the surface, such a simple, natural habit that most of us take it for granted. But, in fact, it is not simple at all. There are many factors, aside from hunger and the need for nutrition, that contribute to our eating patterns.

Food habits are influenced by much more than our own particular likes and dislikes. Culture, religious beliefs, psychological and social attitudes, and the eating habits of our families and friends all play a part. The trend toward more and more households where all the adults work has led to a substantial increase in the use of convenience foods. Very few people have the time to cook everything "from scratch" these days. And so, food merchandisers—with coupons and large amounts of shelf space devoted to snack and convenience foods—influence what goes into the grocery cart and what we eat.

With all these influences (some of them conflicting), how do you choose the best diet? Do you run out and buy every book touting a "new and revolutionary" diet? Do you stick to the four basic food groups that you learned in school? Do you simply eat what you want and not worry about it?

The problem with recommending a diet is that every person is different. The best diet for *you* is the one that makes *you* feel the best. There are certain elements all good diets should contain, and I'll get to those later; but as an overall guiding principle, I offer this advice: choose excellent foods and rely on your common sense to tell you if they are the optimum foods for you.

Listen to your body. Let it guide you to your own best diet. When a food does not suit you, your body will let you know: you may experience abdominal swelling, gas, or a burning sensation in your stomach. You may have headaches or be unusually fatigued. If this happens, contact your physician to determine if you have a food allergy.

The foods you choose will be influenced by your goals and priorities. Obviously, if you weigh 250 pounds, and need to lose a substantial amount of weight, your diet will be different from that of someone who wants to shed a spare 10 pounds. People who do a lot of physical labor will need a different diet from those whose jobs are sedentary. There are as many variables as there are human beings eating. Your Great Legs Profile will show you the factors that you need to consider when choosing your diet.

As a physician I am well aware that there are many conflicting theories in the nutritional advice circulating these days. The study of nutrition has only just begun to receive serious consideration from the medical field. As health professionals continue to do more research in nutrition, new and more accurate information will emerge. I urge you to keep up with advances in nutrition, since it is so important to the way you—and your legs—feel and look. Use your common sense and the basic knowledge in this book to tell you if a particular theory of diet and nutrition would be beneficial to you.

◆ WHAT'S GOOD TO EAT

Approximately forty specific nutrients are presently believed to be needed by the body. These nutrients fall into five general classifications: proteins, carbohydrates, fats, vitamins, and minerals. Every food is composed of varying amounts and combinations of nutrients. No single food contains all the nutrients necessary to maintain good health. Most experts agree that a healthy diet is made up of a combination of foods from each of the five categories.

PROTEINS

Proteins provide the material that builds muscles, so they represent an essential nutrient. In recent years, however, nutritional experts have found that a typical American diet contains too much protein and that our protein is frequently derived from sources that are high in fat and low in fiber, such as full-fat dairy products and red meat. Both red meat and dairy products are good sources of protein, but should not be relied on to meet all your protein needs. Excellent low-fat sources of protein are fish, poultry, legumes, and grains.

CARBOHYDRATES

Carbohydrates are the source of the body's energy. Digestion breaks carbohydrates down into simple sugars that are absorbed into the blood stream and carried to tissues, where energy is released. If the broken-down sugars are not immediately needed, the body converts them into glycogen, which is stored in the muscles and the liver. (That's why runners and other athletes eat lots of carbohydrates before a race or competition; they want to build up their stores of glycogen.) If there is a vast oversupply of broken-down sugars, however, the body converts them into fat.

Simple carbohydrates break down easily, giving you a quick energy boost. Refined sugar is one of the simplest carboydrates. A candy bar does give you a short-lived lift, but if you don't use all that energy, it will be converted to fat.

Complex carboydrates, which contain not only sugars but starch and fiber as well, break down less easily and give the body a long-lasting, steady supply of energy. Whole grains and legumes are the best sources of complex carbohydrates. Fruits and vegetables are also excellent.

FATS

A small amount of fat— about two teaspoons a day— is necessary in a well-balanced diet to provide essential fatty acids. But studies show that the average American consumes far too much fat. Fat is, of course, present in oils, butter, and margarine; but many other foods contain fat as well. These include dairy products, olives, nuts, seeds, and avocados. An excess of fat in the diet is associated with many serious health problems—particularly heart disease, hardening of the arteries, and some types of cancer.

VITAMINS

Vitamins are chemicals our bodies need for growth and development. Our bodies cannot produce vitamins, so we must get them from the food we eat. Each vitamin plays a specific role in the body. There can be no "understudies" where vitamins are concerned; no vitamin can take the part of another.

Certain foods have long been recognized as especially good sources of specific vitamins. Vitamin A, which is vital for maintaining the light-detection mechanism of the eye, is found in carrots, cabbage, and beets. The vitamin B complex, which regulates various functions relating to growth and energy production, is best obtained from whole grains. For vitamin C, which is important for healthy skin and gums, look to citrus fruits, tomatoes, and green peppers. Of course, you can get these vitamins—and others—from many food sources. It is important to eat a variety of good, wholesome foods for adequate vitamin intake.

Vitamin supplements in pill and capsule form are widely available, but most nutritionists would agree that they are not an adequate substitute for a wholesome and well-balanced diet.

MINERALS

The body requires many minerals—some in traces, some in larger amounts—for such essential functions as bone-building, retaining body fluids, and digesting food. Like vitamins, the body cannot produce minerals, so we must get them from our food.

Three of the most important minerals are calcium, iron, and potassium. Calcium is found in milk and dairy products, leafy green vegetables (especially romaine lettuce, collards, and watercress), and shellfish. For iron there are liver, spinach, raisins, and Swiss chard. Look for potassium in bananas, sweet potatoes, and melons.

Of course, the foods I've mentioned here are not the only sources of protein, carbohydrates, fats, vitamins, and minerals. There are many, many good food sources for all these essential nutrients. The more kinds of foods you include in your diet, the better balanced it is likely to be.

Although I can't prescribe the right diet for *you*, I can give you these guidelines. Choose foods that are:

- low in fat
- low in sugar
- low in salt
- high in complex carbohydrates
- whole and unrefined

Basically this means giving up fatty, sugary, salty foods and choosing whole grains and cereals, fresh fruits and vegetables, legumes, fish, poultry, and low-fat dairy products.

◆ TEN BASIC PRINCIPLES FOR GOOD EATING

Even though there are many areas on which nutritional experts do not agree, there are ten basic principles that few would dispute.

1. DRINK LOTS OF WATER.

Drink water (six to eight glasses a day) before and between meals. A glass of water taken one hour before a meal will fill your stomach and calm your appetite. Then, you will eat more slowly, digest better, and get more value and pleasure from the food you eat.

If you are troubled by constipation (which creates pressure that inhibits lymph and vein drainage and can cause your legs to swell), try this: when you get up in the morning, drink one glass of cold water. Wait for five minutes, then drink one glass of hot water. The laxative effect is immediate.

2. CUT OUT CAFFEINE.

"But I only drink one cup of coffee a day." And how many cups of tea, how many colas, how much chocolate? Add up all those doses of caffeine and you have given your body a powerful jolt it doesn't need. Caffeine has many unwanted effects, but in terms of your legs it can dilate veins and raise blood pressure.

Decaffeinated coffee (unless it has been decaffeinated by the water-process method) is not a good alternative: the treatment to remove the caffeine includes the use of arsenic! Herbal teas make lovely hot drinks, particularly because different teas have different properties—mint is stimulating, chamomile calming, and so forth. Many restaurants now offer herbal teas. You can always carry a teabag or two in your purse, and make your own herbal tea wherever hot water is available.

3. REDUCE YOUR SALT INTAKE.

Salt in minute quantities is required by the body. However, it occurs naturally in many foods; and you will get all the salt you need by eating a well-balanced diet. Salt contributes to the fluid retention that brings on swollen ankles, aching or heavy legs, and loss of shape and definition of the legs.

Watch for hidden sources of salt: cheese, anchovies, olives, pickles, potato chips, and other "munchies." All soft drinks, except seltzer water, contain salt. Those "diet" drinks you may have been guzzling are not very good for your diet.

Many canned and convenience foods also contain an excess of added salt. For example, one-half cup of fresh green beans contains 3 milligrams of salt; one-half cup of canned beans can have over 300 milligrams of salt. One teaspoon of salt contains 2000 milligrams; the National Academy of Science dietary guidelines recommend a limit of 1100 to 3300 milligrams of salt per day.

4. ELIMINATE REFINED SUGAR.

White sugar contains *not one* of the more than forty essential nutrients. And yet a typical American gets about 25 percent of his or her calories from sugar. Talk about empty calories! Learn to satisfy your sweet tooth with fresh fruit. Your body and your legs will love you for it.

5. MAKE DIETARY FAT YOUR ENEMY.

The relationship between a high-fat diet and your body is very simple. If you eat more fat than your body can use (and fat burns very slowly compared to carbohydrates), your body will store the unused portion on your legs—or elsewhere on your body.

The worst fats are those classified as saturated (those that harden at room temperature). Look for saturated fats in meats, cheese, chocolate, lard and beef suet, and palm and coconut oil. Read labels carefully: palm and coconut oil are widely present in such junk food as potato chips and in precooked convenience foods. Although cheese is a good source of calcium, it has a very high fat content. Avoid all deep-fried foods.

To get the fat you need each day, rely on cold-pressed virgin olive oil. The fat in certain fatty fish—salmon, tuna, mackerel, bluefish, trout—has been shown to contain substances that are believed to protect against heart disease. Olives, nuts, seeds, and avocados are also high in fats, so be sure to eat these in moderation.

6. AVOID ALCOHOL.

Alcoholic beverages have no nutritive value, so consuming them means consuming empty calories. One of the many things alcohol does to the body is dilate veins, so you can easily see why it is undesirable in terms of your legs. Of course, an occasional drink or glass of wine will not ruin either your diet or your legs; but do use your common sense when it comes to drinking alcohol.

7. EAT QUALITY (COMPLEX) CARBOHYDRATES.

A diet based largely on whole grains and cereals and fresh fruits and vegetables ensures you a steady supply of energy. After a meal rich in complex carbohydrates you will feel more satisfied and less inclined to snack on fatty, sugary, and salty foods. Reaching and maintaining your optimum weight is easy on a high-carbohydrate diet. The more good food you give your body, the more good food it will crave. You will automatically cut out junk foods and change the vicious cycle of dieting into a nutritious cycle of good eating and good health.

8. EAT SUFFICIENT BUT NOT EXCESSIVE AMOUNTS OF PROTEIN.

Protein is absolutely essential for well-developed muscular legs and strong blood vessel walls. The typical American diet, however, contains too much protein. In her *Good Food Book*, Jane Brody recommends that adults age 19 and above eat 0.36 grams of protein per pound of body weight. If you weigh 120 pounds, you will need about 43 grams of protein per day.

That may seem like a lot of protein, but if your diet relies heavily on meat, it is very easy to get that much—and more—in one day. Let me give you some figures. A 3.5 ounce serving of lean, broiled beef contains about 24 grams of protein, or half your daily allowance if you weigh 120 pounds. By contrast, 3.5 ounces of cooked white beans contains only about 8 grams of protein.

Meat, poultry, seafood, eggs, and dairy products are complete proteins; they contain all the essential amino acids necessary for the body's full use of a protein food. Grains, cereals, legumes (beans and peas), nuts, and seeds are incomplete proteins; they all lack at least one essential amino acid. You can combine incomplete proteins to make them complete. Jane Brody's simple rules are: combine any legume with any grain, nut, or seed; combine any incomplete protein with small amounts of a complete protein.

9. GET YOUR ESSENTIAL VITAMINS AND MINERALS.

Vitamin and mineral deficiencies can cause any number of problems for your legs. Lack of dietary iron causes your feet to feel cold and your legs to tire easily with exercise. A rash on your thighs that looks like permanent goose bumps signals a deficiency of vitamin A. A diet low in calcium and magnesium causes leg muscles to twitch intermittently or to cramp after exercise or during the night. And a diet that lacks sufficient zinc and manganese causes ligaments to become overly loose, predisposing ankles or knees to injury.

10. EAT A VARIETY OF HIGH-FIBER FOODS.

Food fiber is the part of a food that remains wholly or partly undigested by the body's natural intestinal juices. Whole grains and cereals, bran, legumes, fruits, and vegetables are all excellent sources of fiber.

Without adequate food fiber and the bulk it provides, your intestines are not stimulated to contract properly, and therefore your body wastes can't move efficiently through your system. You become constipated, which, as I've said, is not good for your legs.

If your Great Legs Profile shows that your eating habits are way out of line with the ten dietary principles I've just outlined, then it is time to change your eating habits. Changing habits is not always easy, so here are a few hints to help you get out of a vicious cycle and into a nutritious cycle.

♦ *Understand and accept your present eating habits.*

Identify the needs your eating habits satisfy, then consider alternative ways to satisfy those needs. For example, if you eat to cheer yourself up when you're feeling down, choose an activity other than eating that would satisfy you—taking a walk, seeing a movie, listening to music, and so forth.

♦ *Use visualization techniques.*

In a quiet place where you can relax, vividly picture your new eating habits. Use all your senses to create a mental image of how you will look and feel when you have acquired these new habits. As your unconscious accepts this new picture of yourself, you will find it easier to change and stick to your new eating habits.

♦ *Seek appropriate support.*

Do not hesitate to call on help when you need it—from a friend, family member, or a medical professional or therapist.

Always keep in mind that your new eating habits will serve you well in the long run. You have far more to gain than healthier, more attractive legs. You are creating a healthier, more attractive you: a body and a state of mind that will go the distance.

5

LIMBER LIMBS

How

exercise

affects

your

legs;

what

exercises

to do

for

them.

A lifelong program of sensible exercise will do great things for your Great Legs. Active muscles are attractive muscles! But even more important, an active person is an attractive person. That is, of course, the hidden benefit of all exercise. When you increase your energy through exercise, it shows. And not only in the great shape of your legs, but also in the rest of your body. You become attractive in the simplest sense of the word: you attract other people.

As you have no doubt been told many times, you should always consult a physician before beginning any exercise program. Discuss with your doctor your exercise goals, how you came to establish your priorities, and your timetable for achieving them. If your doctor advises you for any reason to forego or modify certain routines, take heart. Improving your overall health is, after all, one of the primary objectives of any exercise program. What good are shapelier legs if you have achieved them at the risk of aggravating a preexisting physical condition?

A final caveat. If one of your Great Legs Goals is to lose weight, don't take too seriously the numbers you see on the scale. Look at your body's shape to see if your exercise routine is paying off. Muscle fiber weighs more than fat, so when you exercise you lose fat and build muscle. Your weight may stay the same or even increase. Your body contour, however, changes (for the better!) and you're in superior overall physical condition.

Exercise comes in two types: aerobic and muscle-specific. **Aerobic exercise** improves the cardiovascular system in your legs—and your overall cardiovascular system—and replaces fat tissue with muscle tissue. **Muscle-specific exercises** shape your legs by working and strengthening particular muscles or muscle groups. A smart exercise program includes both types.

◆ AEROBIC EXERCISE

Aerobic exercise improves your heart rate, respiration, and circulation. Your heart is strengthened by pumping at a faster, more demanding rate, and your lungs expand by working harder to take in more oxygen. More oxygen is moving through your body at a faster rate, thereby improving your circulation. And as I've said before, good circulation is critically important for healthy, attractive legs.

Aerobic exercise also burns energy (calories), so you may lose weight. But remember, you first burn the calories from carbohydrates in the muscle tissue. You don't begin to burn stored fat until you have used up your available carbohydrates, which include the glycogen stored in your muscles.

The final benefit of aerobic exercise is endurance: you can exercise for longer periods and with greater intensity without tiring. This endurance does not end with your exercise period — you will find you have more energy for the rest of the things you do, too.

Aerobic exercise is any steady, sustained exercise that raises your heart and respiration rates. Walking, running, bicycling, swimming, rowing, and jumping rope are all aerobic exercise. So is aerobics, or aerobic dancing, the organized dance and exercise workouts that are so popular these days.

MINDING THE SPEED LIMIT

WARNING: During aerobic exercise you should never feel out of breath and you should *never exceed your target heart rate*.

Here's how to determine your target heart rate:

First, calculate *your* maximum heart rate. Subtract your age from a base figure of 220 beats per minute for women and 205 beats per minute for men. That figure is *your* maximum heart rate. For instance, a 40-year-old woman will have a maximum heart rate of 180 beats per minute.

Next, take a percentage of your maximum heart rate to arrive at your target heart rate. Beginners should start to work at a target rate of 50 percent; as you advance, gradually increase your target rate to between 60 and 80 percent of your maximum heart rate.

For example, a 40-year-old woman just beginning an exercise program will work to 50 percent of her maximum rate of

180 beats per minute. Therefore, her target heart rate is 90 beats per minute. As she increases her endurance, she can raise that rate to 108 to 144 beats per minute. No matter how fit she becomes, she should *never* exceed 144 beats per minute, and she should never even reach 180 beats per minute.

The easiest way to gauge your heart rate is to take the pulse of your carotid artery. Place your index and third finger lightly on the left side of your neck, just below your jaw bone. You should feel a pulsing sensation. (If you have trouble locating the exact spot, trace a path slightly down and then forward of your earlobe.) Using a clock or watch with a sweep second hand, count the number of pulses for 6 seconds. Multiply the number of pulses by 10. This will give you your heart rate per minute.

Remember to start slowly and increase your target heart rate gradually. You can increase your heart rate by increasing the duration of the exercise, the intensity of the exercise (run faster, map out a cycling route with more hills), or the frequency of the exercise (work out more times per week).

You should always be able to carry on a conversation during an aerobic exercise. If you can't, slow down; you are overdoing it. Breathlessness is one sign that you have gone beyond your target heart rate. When you do that, you put your body in an *anaerobic* state; that is, you're not supplying enough oxygen to your muscles. You could experience cramps and may even damage your muscles. So, I repeat, never exceed your target heart rate.

WARM UP AND COOL DOWN

No matter what type of exercise you choose, you must always warm up and stretch your muscles before you start. (It is a good idea to do some stretching exercises every day, whether or not you work out as well.) You must raise your heart rate gradually and prime your muscles for exercise. If you jump right in to vigorous exercise you can injure your muscles and joints.

After exercise you must cool down and stretch again, gradually lowering your heart rate and restretching the muscles, which contract during exercise.

Before a workout, warm up by walking in place, gradually increasing your heart rate by raising your knees higher and swinging your arms further forward and back. Make sure your movements are smooth, not jerky. Then stretch all your muscles, paying particular attention to the muscles you will be using. Stretching exercises also give your body flexibility and lend grace to your movements.

Always stretch without bouncing and hold each movement for about 5 to 6 seconds (more if you are comfortable doing so). You should feel the stretch in your muscles, but you should never feel pain. If you stretch to the point of pain, you may tear muscle or tendon fibers.

After your workout, never stop exercising abruptly. Wind down slowly, progressively coming to a full stop. Because your heart has pumped a tremendous amount of blood to your legs during exercise, a sudden stop can prevent the blood from getting back into general circulation and reaching the brain, causing you to feel dizzy or faint. Stretch again, then take a moment to relax fully and feel the wonderful effects of your workout.

You will find an excellent set of pre- and post-stretches on pages 85 and 100.

CHOOSING YOUR AEROBIC EXERCISE

Any aerobic activity is beneficial to your legs; but because each activity uses different muscle groups, the effect on your legs will be different. No matter which aerobic exercise you choose, however, make sure it is one you enjoy. If you don't enjoy the activity, you will be less likely to stick to your exercise program.

AEROBIC DANCING classes are offered practically everywhere now—in health clubs, community centers, aerobic dance studios, and television exercise programs. You can also buy records, video cassettes, and audio cassettes for your own home workouts. Aerobic dancing gives you a good cardiovascular workout, as well as exercising specific muscles. It's also a lot of fun, which is why so many people have chosen it. Be aware, however, that aerobic dancing can cause knee injuries and shin splints. Because of this, many aerobic workouts have been modified. When you choose a workout, make sure it is one of the newer, low-impact routines.

It is best to do aerobics on a floor that "gives": wood, carpeted, or elevated. Concrete, cement, marble, or basement floors that sit directly on a foundation make for a harder impact on your legs. Floors without any "give" are often the cause of shin splints—sharp pains in the outer calf muscle caused by muscle tearing away from the bone. You can guard against shin splints by carefully warming up before you exercise and by putting your heel down with each movement. If you do get shin splints, rest and switch to a nonimpact aerobic exercise such as walking, bicycling, or swimming until your condition improves.

Investing in a good pair of shoes will also lessen the possibility of injury. The shoes should fit comfortably and be well-cushioned. The toe box should be roomy enough to accommodate lateral movement of the foot. Running shoes are not good for aerobic dancing because they are designed to accommodate forward motion of the foot. Replace your shoes frequently; don't work out in old beat-up shoes. That is penny-wise and pound-foolish.

WALKING is a sport almost anyone can enjoy. Unlike running, it causes very few injuries. To achieve aerobic benefit, however, you must walk at a pace of at least 4 miles per hour for forty-five minutes to an hour. A 120-pound woman will burn 230 calories per hour at this rate. You can make walking more productive by pumping your arms or by carrying half-pound wrist or hand weights. This "fitness walking" is especially good for the muscles in your thighs and in your derrière.

PERFORMANCE (RACE) WALKING increases walking speed to between 4-1/2 and 6 miles per hour. Because the muscles in your legs were not made to walk this fast, performance walking actually taxes your body more than running. That same 120-pound woman can burn about 500 calories per hour with performance walking. If you have not been exercising regularly, performance walking is *not* the place to begin. You must build strength and endurance before taking on this taxing activity.

Performance walking is not just walking faster; it requires a special form. Your right heel strikes the ground directly in front of the big toe of your left foot and vice versa. Your arms are bent at the elbow and pump vigorously as you walk. Your body leans slightly forward from the ankles but does not bend at the waist. Rotating your hip forward and down as your leg moves forward lengthens your stride.

No matter what type of walking you choose, you must have good shoes. They should be somewhat stiff across the instep and flexible across the toe joints. The shoes should fit your heel firmly. They should also be made of leather and have tiny holes for ventilation. To test the fit of your shoes (when you are wearing them), run your thumb across the top from your big toe to your little toe. You should feel a gentle wave of ripples.

RUNNING (JOGGING) can get your legs in shape in short order, but not everyone can withstand the high impact running imposes on the bones and joints of the feet, ankles, and back. If running agrees with you, by all means do it; but if you find yourself with frequent joint and muscle aches, reconsider your choice. Remember: *never* run without stretching both before and after.

Again, good running shoes are crucial for avoiding injury. They should have a firm, stable heel. Your foot should not lift out of the shoe. The whole shoe, but especially the heel, should be well-cushioned to reduce stress on the Achilles tendon. To allow for forward motion there should be one-half inch between the tip of your longest toe and the forward end of the shoe. The toe box should be wide enough to allow your toes to spread on impact.

BICYCLING burns between 400 and 600 calories an hour during a vigorous ride. It is an excellent aerobic activity. Beware, however, that biking builds the quadriceps more than it builds the hamstrings. This can cause bulging thighs. It can also affect your posture by causing you to sway forward (in order to compensate for the relative underdevelopment of your hamstrings and the peroneal muscles in your calves). Women who frequently wear high heels often have this same type of muscle imbalance, and therefore do not have the most well-shaped legs.

If you choose bicycling, remember to supplement this quadriceps-building activity with muscle-specific exercises that will work the other muscles in your legs.

SWIMMING, besides being a top-notch cardiovascular exercise, also tones the legs well. Because the water supports the body during exercise, swimming is a low-impact and low-injury sport. Many swimmers find working out in the water especially relaxing.

ROWING benefits the cardiovascular system and is good exercise if you want to work your upper body muscles as well as your legs. Beware, however, that, like bicycling, it exercises mainly the quadriceps muscles and can leave you with over-developed thighs unless you add muscle-specific exercises to work the other leg muscles.

DANCING can be a fun-filled route to well-shaped legs of mixed-fiber type. Ballet creates the leanest legs, as almost all the movements build slow-twitch muscle fiber. Tap dancing is the most fast-twitch activity. Square dancing, folk dancing, ballroom, Jazzercise, and interpretive or modern dance fall somewhere in between. The aerobic value of dancing varies with the type you choose, but, in general, dancing does not build endurance as well as activities in which movement is steady and sustained.

TENNIS and other **RACKET SPORTS** are played with rapid movements that promote fast-twitch fiber growth. On women who already have a preponderance of fast-twitch muscles, tennis and racket sports can readily build up the thighs. The aerobic value of the racket sports depends a lot on your level of play. Because these are "stop-and-start" sports, in general they do not build endurance as well as the steadier, sustained-movement activities.

GOLF is beneficial *only* if you walk the course. Even if you walk the course, however, you stop and start frequently and so do not derive the same aerobic benefit you would from uninterrupted walking at even 3 miles per hour.

◆ MUSCLE-SPECIFIC EXERCISES

To build specific muscles and muscle groups, I recommend the #11 Workout (by One Better, Inc.) developed by fitness specialist Pauline S. Molt. The workout is called #11 because doing it regularly is supposed to give you a score one better than Bo Derek's "10." The exercises presented here are a portion of the total body #11 Workout.

Pauline Molt's program is a balanced muscle workout that stresses correct body alignment, proper body mechanics, and exercising at one's own level of physical capability. It is suitable for beginners, for those who need to restore muscle tone after bed rest, and for the severely overweight. It also works for seasoned exercisers who want to shape and tone their legs.

Since everyone's needs are different, there is no single magic formula that will determine the frequency, intensity, and duration of your muscle-specific exercise program. I can, however, give you some guidelines for adapting the exercises to your own needs:

If you are a beginner, perform the whole workout, but start with only as many repetitions of each exercise as you can *comfortably* perform. As you build strength, gradually increase the number of repetitions, remembering always to stay inside *your* comfort zone. Try to exercise at least three times per week. Increase that to four or even five times a week if you are comfortable doing so. Don't overdo it. Learn to listen to your body. It will tell you when to try harder and when to rest.

For **muscle tone after bed rest**, select only one exercise for each muscle group. If you feel comfortable with only one or two repetitions of that exercise, fine. Increase repetitions and add exercises as you are able to do so.

Severely overweight persons *must* combine these exercises with a nutrition program and aerobic conditioning. Walking is the best aerobic exercise for the severely overweight. As you lose fat and build muscle, increase the speed and duration of your walking. Start slowly with the muscle-specific exercises, doing only as many exercises and repetitions as you are able to do without strain. As you trim down and gain strength and endurance, slowly increase the number of exercises and repetitions.

People who are **somewhat overweight or flabby** from lack of muscle tone should try to do the exercises three or four times per week. These exercises develop lean muscle mass in the legs while reducing the percentage of fat in them. If you do the exercises faithfully, the results will soon become visible.

To **maintain shape and tone**, do the exercises a minimum of three times a week.

Try not to exercise three days in a row and then rest for four days. Exercise every other day or two days in a row followed by one day of rest. Steady, regular exercise will be more beneficial than sudden bursts of exercise with long rest periods in between.

If you wish to do more than maintain shape and tone, wearing ankle weights will increase the work for your legs. The additional weight resistance develops greater contour and definition in your muscles. A word of warning, though: if you take up weight-resistance training, be sure to do so with the help of a qualified instructor. Instruction on correct body alignment and positioning is necessary if you are to avoid joint injuries.

You can also use weight-resistance machines, such as the Nautilus system. These systems isolate the action of individual muscles to build size and shape. The weight resistance must be increased as muscle strength develops. Again, it is important to work with a qualified instructor to set up a program and ensure that you are using the machines correctly.

BEFORE YOU BEGIN

Here are some important things to remember while performing the exercises:

1. Breathe normally during exercise. Never hold your breath. You should be able to carry on a conversation while exercising. If you can't, you are overdoing it.

2. Work your muscles to the point of slight discomfort but *never* to the point of pain.

3. Hold in your abdominal muscles firmly at all times to support your lower back.

4. Move smoothly and consistently, without any abrupt jerking or kicking.

5. Perform the prescribed releasing action after each exercise. When you pause and relax after working a muscle you quickly become attuned to the capabilities of that muscle. Many people find they can comfortably continue to work the muscle after releasing.

6. Pay close attention to correct body positioning by using the diagrams that accompany each exercise.

7. Stretch, never bounce, in the stretching exercises.

8. Exercise to music that has a medium, even beat.

9. Work on a firm, padded surface, such as carpeting or an exercise mat.

10. Make sure your upper body is relaxed and in a comfortable position so that you can concentrate on working your legs. Hold your head straight: your chin should not drop or point toward the ceiling.

THE #11 WORKOUT

Now, let's turn on the music and warm up by walking in place. Increase the intensity of the warm-up by raising your knees higher and swinging your arms forward and back in controlled movements. When your muscles feel warm and supple, begin the pre-stretch exercises. Hold the pre-stretch positions for about 5 to 6 seconds each—longer if you feel comfortable doing so.

Pre-Stretches

Calf Stretch [Figure 1]

With arms outstretched, place your palms against a wall. Your feet should be parallel and a hip-width apart. Gently bend your elbows and lean in toward the wall. Keep your back straight, not rounded or arched, and your heels flat on the floor.

Quadriceps Stretch [Figure 2]

Place your left hand against a wall or other firm support. Keeping the left knee bent, grasp your right ankle with your right hand and pull your foot up toward your derrière. Feel the stretch in your right thigh as you hold the position. Stretch only as far as you can without pain. Repeat with the left leg.

Hamstrings Stretch [Figure 3]

Sit on the floor with your legs straight in front of you. With your arms outstretched, flex your feet and bend forward from the hips. Feel the stretch in the back of your thighs. Keep your head up and back straight. (When you first begin to do this stretch, your arms may not reach out over your toes, as in the diagram. As you gain flexibility, however, your arms will not only reach your toes but will pass beyond them.)

Inner Thigh Stretch [Figure 4]

Still sitting on the floor, spread your legs wide (but only as far as they will comfortably go). Flex your feet, keep your knees loose (unlocked), and bend forward from the hips, placing your palms flat on the floor in front of you. Keep your elbows bent and your back straight. As you become more flexible, your legs will spread wider and your chest will move closer to the floor.

Now that you're warmed up and stretched, you're ready to start your workout. Remember to keep your abdominal muscles held in firmly for all the exercises.

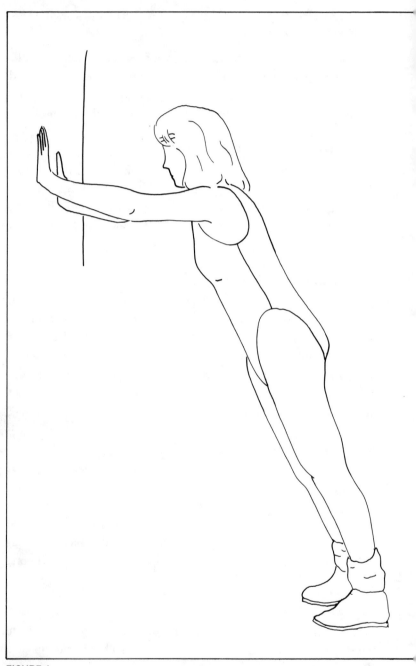

FIGURE 1

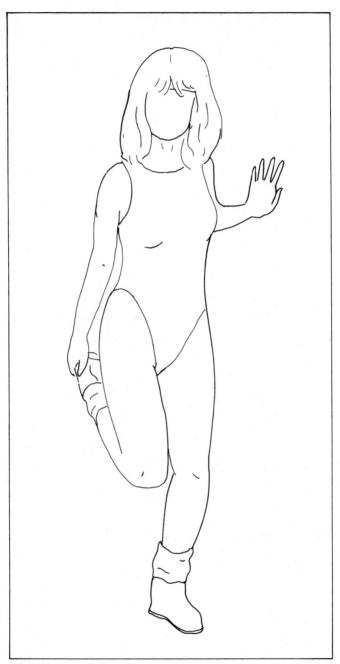

FIGURE 2

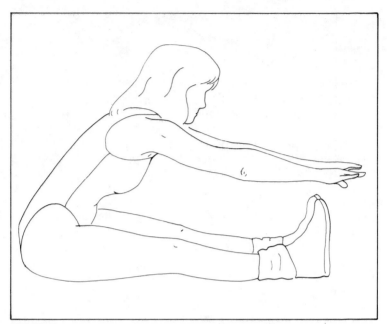

FIGURE 3

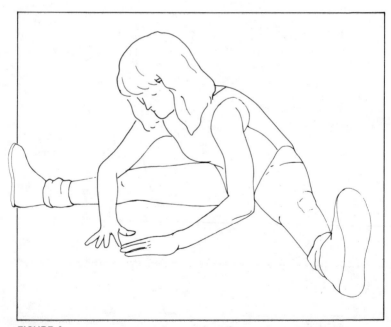

FIGURE 4

Quadriceps Exercises

1. With feet a hip-width apart and parallel [Figure 5] and knees bent, raise and lower the hips, using the front thigh muscles. Keep your back straight (not rounded over or arched) while the thigh muscles raise and lower your hips. To release, return to a standing position, then bend the knees alternately.

2. Lie on your back [Figure 6] and raise your upper body, supporting yourself on your bent elbows. Keep the abdominals held firmly. Bend your left leg. With the foot flexed, raise and lower your right leg. Do an equal number of repetitions with the foot pointed. Release the muscle by bending and extending your right leg. Then switch legs, bending the right and working the left. Release the left leg before going on to the next exercise.

Hamstrings Exercise [Figure 7]

Kneel down, supporting your upper body on your bent elbows, palms on the floor. With the foot flexed, raise and lower your right leg behind you. Do an equal number of repetitions with the foot pointed. Then, straighten the right leg and raise and lower it, first with the foot flexed and then with the foot pointed.

To release, alternate bending and extending the leg. Then assume the position in Figure 8. Sit back on your heels and extend your arms straight in front of you, palms on the floor. This position relaxes the supporting knee and stretches the body.

Repeat the hamstring exercise and release on the left side.

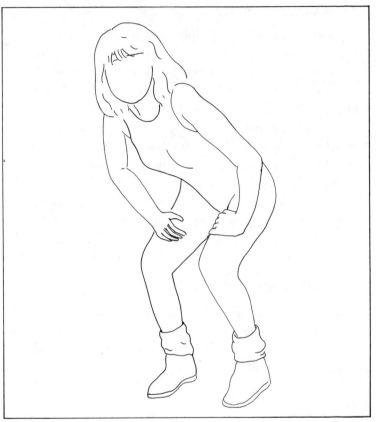

FIGURE 5

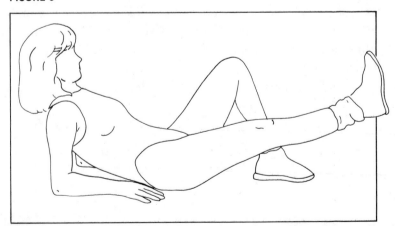

FIGURE 6

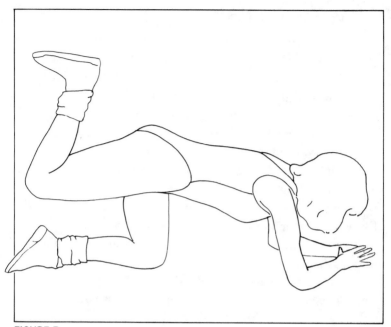

FIGURE 7

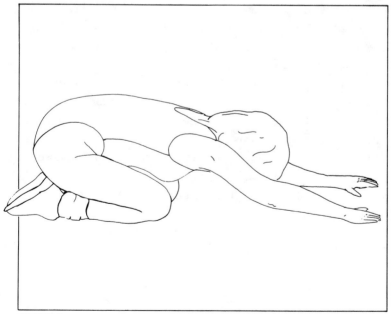

FIGURE 8

Outer Thigh Exercises

1. Lie on your left side [Figure 9], supporting your upper body on your bent left elbow. Bend and draw in your knees so that your thighs are at a right angle to your body. Raise and lower the right (top) leg with the foot flexed, then with the foot pointed. Release by bending and extending the working leg.

2. Lie on your left side [Figures 10, 11], left arm extended (palm down), head resting on the extended arm. Bend your right elbow and place your right palm flat on the floor. Bend your left leg so that your thigh is at a right angle to your body. Extend your right (top) leg so that it too is at a right angle to your body. Raise and lower the right leg, first with the foot flexed, then with the foot pointed. Release by bending and extending the working leg.

Remain in the same position, but extend your right (top) leg down, keeping your body in one long line. Raise and lower the right leg, first with the foot flexed, then with the foot pointed. Bend and extend the working leg to release.

3. Release by rolling onto your back [Figures 12, 13, 14], knees bent, feet on the floor. With both hands clasp your right leg and draw it toward your chest. Then, holding onto the calf or thigh (never the knee) extend the right leg. Keep the knee loose, not locked. In this position you may flex and point your toes and/or circle your ankles inward and outward. Finish by drawing both knees into your chest with both hands clasped around your legs. Do this release after you have completed all three inner thigh exercises (or as many as you have chosen if you are on an abbreviated program).

4. Repeat the exercise(s), working the left leg. Release the left leg.

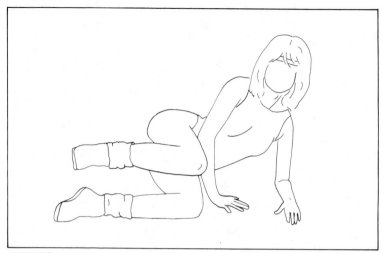

FIGURE 9

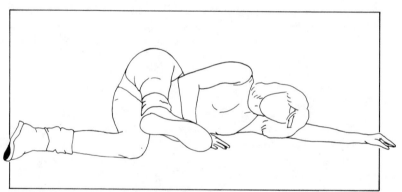

FIGURE 10

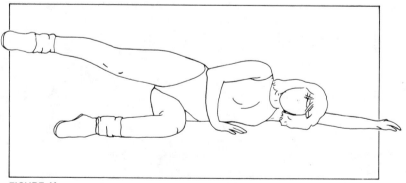

FIGURE 11

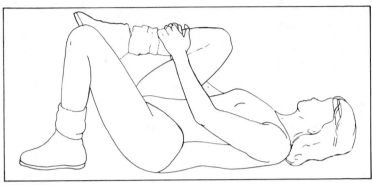

FIGURE 12

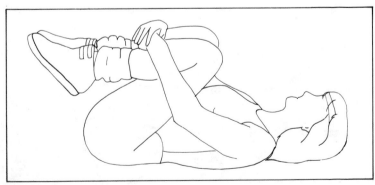

FIGURE 13

FIGURE 14

Inner Thigh Exercises

1. Lie on your left side [Figure 15], left arm extended (palm down), head resting on the extended arm. Bend your right elbow and place your right palm on the floor. Bend your right (top) leg so that your thigh is at a right angle to your body. Allow your right knee to rest on the floor. Raise and lower your left (bottom) leg, first with the foot flexed, then with the foot pointed. To release, bend and extend the left leg. Switch sides and repeat the exercise, working the right leg.

2. Lie on your back [Figures 16, 17], arms bent at the elbows, hands resting (palm up) on the floor. Pressing your lower back into the floor, raise your knees to your chest, then spread them out to the side. Extend your legs as far as you can while still keeping your lower back in contact with the floor. If you must keep your legs fully bent, fine. If you can extend them, keep the knees loose, not locked.

Once you are in position, draw your legs together and apart (without letting them touch), first with feet flexed, then with feet pointed.

3. To release [Figure 18], put the soles of your feet together. Clasp your feet with your hands and gently draw them toward your body.

Calf and Ankle Exercises

1. With your feet a hip-width apart and parallel [Figures 19, 20, 21, 22], raise and lower your heels. Keep your knees loose (not locked). For better balance, place your hands lightly on your thighs. Repeat with toes turned inward, then with toes turned outward. To release, stand on flat feet and bend your knees alternately.

2. With feet a hip-width apart and parallel [Figure 23], bend your knees and place your hands on the floor. Raise your heels. With heels raised, lift and lower your hips. Remember never to bring your hips lower than your knees. To release, alternate bending your knees.

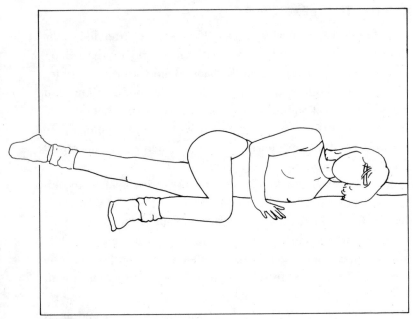

FIGURE 15

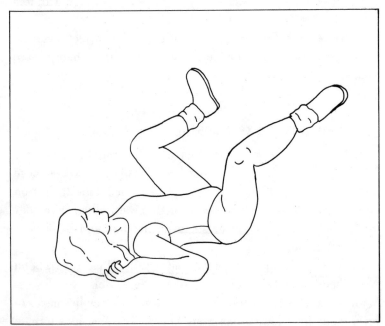

FIGURE 16

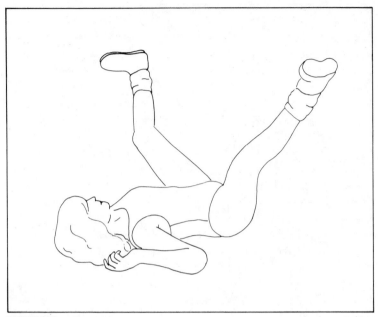

FIGURE 17

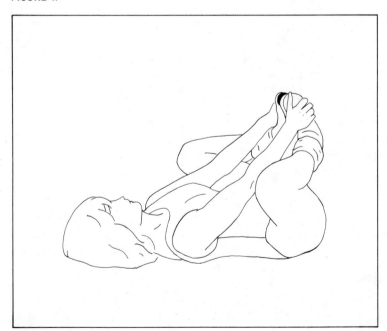

FIGURE 18

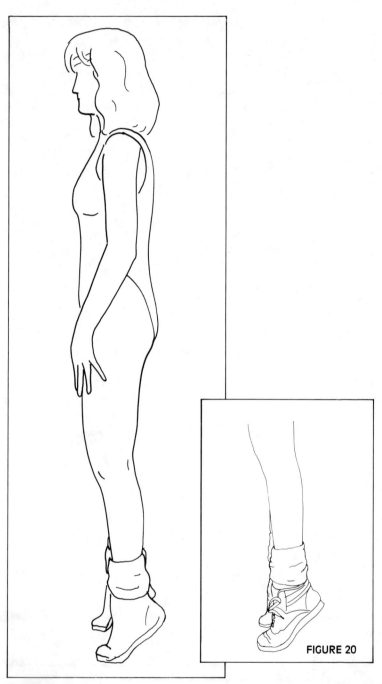

FIGURE 19

FIGURE 20

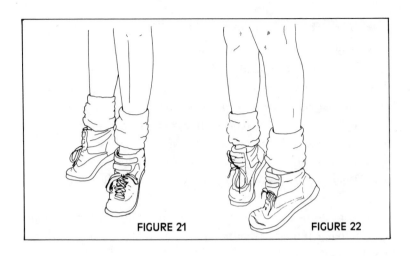

FIGURE 21   FIGURE 22

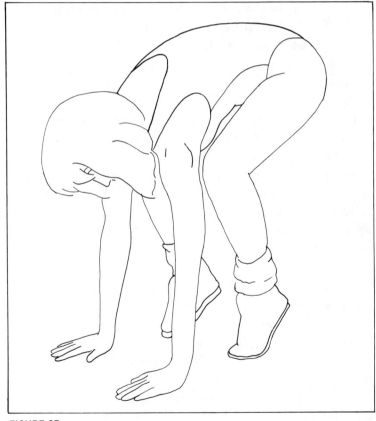

FIGURE 23

Post-Stretch Exercise Sequence

Stretching after you work out is as important as stretching before exercise. Remember, the muscles you've just used have been contracted and need to be lengthened. Also, the body is warm after exercising and the muscles more flexible. So this is an especially good time to stretch. Stretching creates a graceful, well-tuned body. It also relaxes the mind.

These post-stretch exercises may be too advanced for some of you. If so, repeat the pre-stretch exercises until you are stronger and more flexible.

The post-stretch sequence should be done as one smooth, continuous exercise. Breathe deeply and hold in your abdominal muscles firmly.

Stand with your feet about two hip-widths apart [Figure 24]. Roll down slowly, starting from the head and bending each successive vertebra until your hands are resting on the floor. Keep the feet parallel and knees loose. Feel the stretch on the back of the thighs.

Now [Figure 25], slowly "walk" your feet wider by turning out first your toes then your heels until your legs are as wide as is comfortable. In the final position, make your feet parallel and keep the knees loose. Feel the stretch in the inner thigh.

Increase the stretch [Figure 26] by bending your knees alternately.

Walk your toes and heels inward [Figure 27] until your feet are together, then step back with the right leg. Keep your right heel on the floor. Feel the stretch in your right calf and hamstring.

Increase the stretch [Figure 28] by lifting the right heel off the ground and sliding the right foot back as far as it can comfortably go. As you slide the right foot back, bend the left knee deeper and let your body weight come forward over the left knee. Make sure to keep the left knee directly over the left toes and the left heel on the floor. Feel the stretch in your quads.

Pull the right foot in, keeping the knees bent, until your feet are together. Then straighten your legs and step back with the

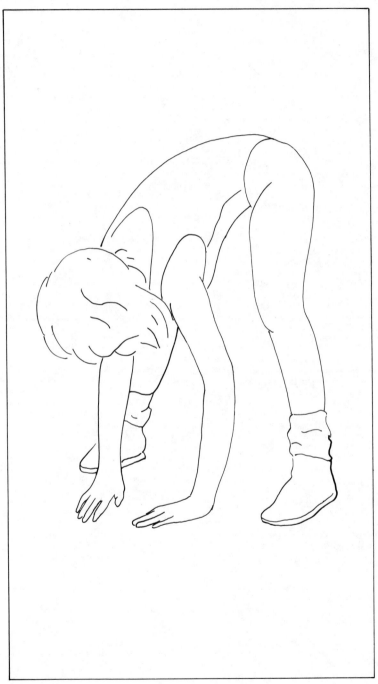

FIGURE 24

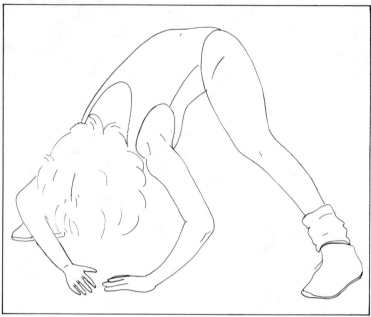

FIGURE 25

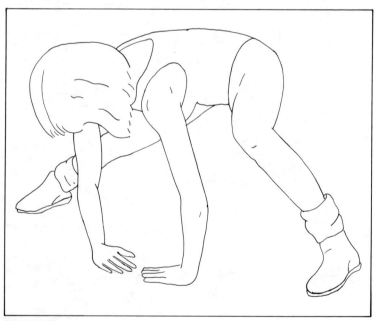

FIGURE 26

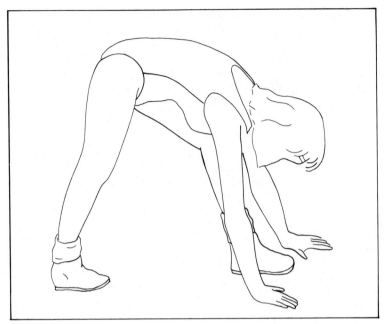

FIGURE 27

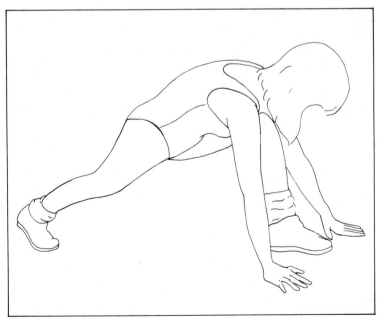

FIGURE 28

left leg and stretch the left calf and hamstring. Increase the stretch on the left side by sliding the left foot back and stretching over the right knee.

To return to standing, keep the right knee bent and pull in the left leg until your feet are together. Keeping the knees slightly bent, slowly roll up, one vertebra at a time.

Congratulations! You have completed your workout. I know you must feel wonderful—energized, limber, and well on your way to having your own Great Legs.

6

Aye There's The Rub

Massage and other techniques to make you and your legs feel great.

Being manipulated isn't all bad, as anyone who's ever given herself over to the sybaritic delight of a good massage knows. Massage is one of those happy instances in which what feels good is also good *for* you. Massage won't give Great Legs the lifelong benefits of excellent nutrition and commonsense exercise, but it can do wonders for your legs in the short run.

Massage improves the circulatory system by speeding up the rate at which blood flows through your body, thus easing the strain on your heart and increasing the supply of oxygen and nutrients that your blood distributes to the rest of the body.

Massage can also prevent—or at least delay—the formation of cellulite, those unattractive clumps of dimpled fatty deposits that sometimes form on your thighs. (See Chapter 12). One of the causes of cellulite is warped connective tissue; fat collects in the ripples. By stretching the connective tissue, massage improves circulation to the tissue, thus allowing more nutrients to reach it. The connective tissue stays strong and supple; there are no—or at least fewer—ripples to attract and hold fatty deposits.

Finally, massage breaks up that swamp-water congestion in your veins and tissues by pushing lymph through your body. This strengthens your immune system, gets rid of poisonous wastes, and helps slim your legs.

Again, I emphasize, good lymph drainage is essential in slimming your legs. With poor lymph drainage any fat you lose while dieting will be taken by your body from a more accessible area—such as your throat or your arms—rather than from your legs.

Massage has all these medical benefits, plus it relaxes you and feels wonderful. And in the cases of illness or injury that leaves a person immobile, massage can partially compensate for lack of exercise and can help restore tone to weak, flabby muscles.

Is it any wonder that I recommend massage so highy? But what kind of massage? There are many massage techniques and it can be confusing to try to choose among them.

It will help you to remember that there are two basic systems of massage: mechanical and reflex. In the **mechanical systems,** the point that is stroked is directly affected. In **reflex systems,** the point that is stroked produces a reflex reaction at another point in the body. Some massage techniques have their basis in either one system or the other; other techniques combine the two systems.

This is an exciting time in the history of massage. Massage therapists are studying old and new massage methods and synthesizing information to create new techniques. Many of these practitioners take the whole body approach I favor. Because there are so many, I will tell you about only the techniques that are the most popular or the most beneficial to your legs. I hope you will try at least one of them.

The American Massage Therapy Association (AMTA) is an international organization of massage therapists. They will help you locate an appropriate massage therapist in your area.

Before you do get a massage, make sure you have no question in your mind about any aspect of your health. If you do, seek a medical diagnosis first to rule out any serious underlying condition.

◆ SWEDISH MASSAGE

What an invigorating experience! A single half-hour session with a trained professional Swedish masseuse can give your circulatory system a workout equivalent to a 5-mile walk.

The first rule a massage therapist learns is: massage toward the heart. After applying a light oil to your body, the masseuse will begin the *effleurage* strokes. These strokes go toward your heart; they work against gravity to improve blood and lymph circulation.

Another technique of Swedish massage is *pétrissage*. This employs kneading and wringing movements that work on muscle fibers to relieve tension and relax the tight muscles caused by too much standing, too much exercise, tension, or fatigue.

Other Swedish massage strokes include *friction*, deep movements on the tendons and ligaments, and *tapotement*, percussive strokes that stimulate the deep body structures.

Swedish massage is the most readily available massage technique. It is the one to seek if you are feeling tired, tense, and sluggish.

◆ SHIATSU (ACUPRESSURE MASSAGE)

Shi is the Japanese word for finger; *atsu* the word for pressure. In Japan, where Shiatsu was developed, blind people are often trained in the technique. They are frequently considered to be among the best practitioners because of the extreme sensitivity they develop in their fingers.

In Shiatsu, the practitioner applies pressure with the thumb and index finger to particular points in your body and to the pathways—called meridians—along which these points occur.

Energy is thought to travel along these meridians. The pressure points are to the meridians what transformers are to a powerline. Any disturbance or imbalance in the "transformers" can cause a loss of energy throughout the body or within internal organs. By applying pressure to the points and meridians, Shiatsu seeks to restore a clear and balanced energy flow.

Today, you can find trained Shiatsu practitioners in most cities. There are also many weekend workshops where you can learn basic Shiatsu techniques to use on yourself and others. If you feel out of kilter or that your energy is blocked by tension or even pain, a Shiatsu massage will help restore your body to balance and comfort.

◆ SPORTS MASSAGE

Sports massage combines a number of massage techniques to help prevent injuries to athletes and improve their performance. To basic Swedish massage strokes it adds *range of motion* movements to improve the condition of the joints and associated muscles.

It may also include *triggerpoint therapy* (also known as *myotherapy*), which seeks to reduce pain located deep within a muscle at spots called triggerpoints. Pain often radiates up or down from these spots, causing intense discomfort. (Triggerpoints are different from the pressure points of Shiatsu in that they are actually located in the muscle and will vary from person to person, rather than being specific locations along the body's energy-flow lines.)

Triggerpoints develop from accidents or injuries—a broken leg perhaps, or a sprained ankle—and they typically appear after some time has elapsed, sometimes months or years after the original trauma.

Pain from triggerpoints is relieved only by sustained pressure. Triggerpoint therapists use fingers, knuckles, and even elbows to provide the sustained pressure that relieves the pain. Triggerpoints cannot be relieved (and may be aggravated) by quick on-and-off pressure, such as probing around a painful muscle.

◆ LYMPH DRAINAGE (VODDER) MASSAGE

If you have a severe problem with excessive fluid retention you may wish to seek out a practitioner of lymph drainage massage. The Vodder technique was developed because, although effective with veins and capillaries, Swedish massage is ineffective in reducing severe edema (swelling) resulting from poor lymph drainage. I must warn you, however, that a trained Vodder practitioner will be difficult to find in North America; but the extra effort to find one may be worth it if you have lymph drainage problems.

In the Vodder technique, no oil is used, and all the practitioner's movements are feather light, applied in tiny circles with only the gentlest pressure. The sequence of movements and the direction of applied pressure varies according to the condition of your legs. In Germany and France, physicians frequently prescribe lymph drainage massage for its sedative and relaxing powers as well as for its effectiveness in treating edema.

There is another group of techniques that are not strictly massage, but are nonetheless beneficial to your legs in correcting imbalances, promoting circulation, or relieving pain.

◆ APPLIED KINESIOLOGY (AK)

AK is used by physical therapists and physical education specialists to evaluate the function and effectiveness of muscles and to then correct muscle imbalances or weaknesses. It is an effective remedy for all types of leg muscle problems, including athletic injuries.

Although most people realize they are stronger in one arm than the other, they may not also realize that they favor one leg over the other. Putting too much weight on one leg causes the muscles to be more developed, the leg to be larger, and the heels on the shoes to wear unevenly.

AK practitioners test right-left leg imbalance as you did in the Great Legs Profile, by examining your weight distribution on two scales placed side by side. Practioners also isolate each individual muscle to test its function. Each muscle has a test position in which it is isolated and contracted. While the muscle is in the test position, the practitioner applies resistance. A strong muscle remains contracted; a weak muscle gives way.

Muscle weaknesses are then strengthened by pressure applied to reflex points. (These are a different set of points than the ones in Shiatsu or triggerpoint therapy.) These reflex points also relate to specific organs and glands. Stimulating these muscle reflex points also stimulates the organ or gland to which they relate. Conversely, stress or diminished function of a related organ or gland can cause a weakness in the related muscle.

For information on how you can learn and use some of the basic principles of AK, write to: The Touch for Health Foundation, 1174 North Lake Avenue, Pasadena, California, 91104.

◆ NEUROMUSCULAR BODYWORK

This technique consists of specific physical manipulation of muscles, ligaments, and tendons. The purpose of the technique is to restore the balance of the body and to achieve a good structural alignment. The technique is applied most of the time with hands only. It is called bodywork rather than massage because the practitioner's fingers move the muscle back into its original place. Bodywork is most effective in improving posture and relieving neuromuscular pain. Unfortunately, there are not many bodywork practitioners in the United States.

◆ REFLEXOLOGY MASSAGE

In primitive times, when we walked on sand or dirt in bare feet, the soles of our feet were constantly massaged. Now, with shoes and concrete, our feet lose a lot of their contact with a massaging surface. Tired feet can drain the whole body of energy. A reflexology massage can restore energy to a fatigued body, making tired feet and legs feel blissfully light.

Reflexology works on the theory that there is a correlation between painful areas of the body and specific points on the feet. Applying pressure to these points on the feet both restores circulation and relieves tension in the corresponding body part. Classes and self-help books on Reflexology are now widely available.

◆ ACUPUNCTURE

Acupuncturists use the same pressure points as Shiatsu practitioners. Instead of applying pressure, however, to restore energy flow and balance along the meridians, they stimulate the points by needle puncture or moxibustion (the burning of tiny bits of herb mugwort, which causes a deep heating of the point). As acupuncture has been widely accepted in the West, modern technology has invented various replacements for the needle, including electrical stimulation and the cold laser beam. Shiatsu practitioners recommend having an acupuncture treatment at the beginning of each season.

◆ HYDROTHERAPY

Sebastian Kniepp was a frail 18th-century German monk who restored himself to health through cold-water treatments of his own devising. These treatments have withstood the test of time; in Germany today, there are twenty Kniepp clinics at which physicians administer treatment.

Unfortunately, there are no Kniepp clinics in North America, but you can replicate the Kniepp thirty-second lower-body immersion technique at home for relief of tired, aching, or swollen legs. It restores circulation by stimulating veins and lymphatic channels.

Fill your bathtub with cold water and place a dry sheet on the floor beside the tub. Wear a warm sweater, but stay naked below the waist. Quickly step into the tub (the first time is always the worst!) and sit with your legs extended. Stay there thirty seconds. Step out of the tub, wrap your lower body in the sheet and hop into bed under a blanket. Rest in bed for twenty minutes. When you get up your legs will feel wonderful. You will thank the good monk as you go briskly about your business.

No matter what your Great Legs Goals, massage—or one of these related techniques—will help you achieve them. I urge you to take advantage of the benefits of massage regularly. Improved circulation and release of tension lead to lovely legs—and a lovely you.

7

TLC (TENDER LEG CARE)

How to have the smoothest, silkiest legs in town.

We can all use a bit of pampering now and then. And that includes our legs. Of course, the external "treats" we give our legs can never replace the long-term benefits of diet and exercise, nor can they duplicate the physical and spiritual lift of an excellent massage. On the other hand, the results of Tender Leg Care are visible immediately. And treating your legs—and yourself—well can make you feel good from the tips of your toes to the top of your head.

◆ SMOOTHING THE ROUGH SPOTS

Perhaps nowhere else on the body is the skin so often dry, scaly, or flaky, as it is on your legs. Your legs are frequently exposed to irritating fabrics, harsh weather, hot water, and damaging chemicals. They also have fewer oil glands than any other part of your body. So your legs need special care, especially when it comes to moisture.

Let's get one thing clear first: There is no way you can actually add moisture to skin. You can, however, prevent excess evaporation of water from your skin through the judicious use of bath oils and body creams and lotions.

But how do you choose an effective oil, cream, or lotion when there are so very many to choose from? First of all, I recommend staying away from bath salts, mousses, and bubble baths—any bath preparation that contains perfume. Perfumes can cause allergies, irritations, and even vaginitis or cystitis.

A good bath oil will have a base of mineral oil and will be mixed with other hydrating (moisturizing) products. A good lotion or cream will contain mineral oil and one or more of the following: petroleum, white wax, lanolin, poly oil 40 stearate, or urea. Don't be misled by price or popularity; some of the least expensive drugstore brands are among the best. Pick one that you like. The smell (scented or unscented), or the texture (thinner or thicker) does not matter. Make it a pleasant experience.

The best way to use a bath oil is to add it to the water once you are already in the bath. Since your skin is already wet, it will retain the oil better. Make sure to use lukewarm water; hot water opens pores and lets moisture escape, just the opposite of what you are trying to do. When you come out of the tub, don't rub yourself dry; just blot carefully with your towel so the oil stays on your skin. Apply a moisturizing cream or lotion while your skin is still damp, so that it will seal in the moisture.

If you shower or bathe without oil, blot dry when you are finished and apply your cream or lotion while your skin is still moist. For extremely dry skin, the ultimate leg moisturizer is pure petroleum jelly, applied sparingly and massaged into the skin. Pure olive oil, cold-pressed, is good too.

If your skin is extremely dry you should also avoid hot baths, saunas, and excessive sun exposure. Use a sunscreen whenever you go bare-legged in the sun. If your legs remain obdurately dry despite these precautions, consult a dermatologist; he or she will prescribe a hydrating agent that will work for you.

Among the many creams and lotions that are available, you will find some that claim to do more than moisturize your skin. Some promise to ease tired legs, firm flabby thighs and even to reduce your weight.

How effective are these concoctions? The pine extracts found in "tired leg" lotions do have a temporary cooling and soothing effect. Firming creams that contain such herbal diuretics as ivy and juniper have only a minimal effect on your skin; but those that contain elastin and collagen can help your skin to hold more water.

Avoid strong deodorant soaps; the chemicals in these soaps can be drying to your skin. Choose instead a superfatted soap that will help retain moisture.

Dry-brushing your legs with a loofah sponge or natural-bristle (*not* nylon) brush is an effective way to keep your skin smooth and to stimulate circulation to the skin on your legs. This brushing removes dead surface skin cells that dehydrate and dry your skin. It also breaks up the accumulations of dead skin that appear in some people as hard whitish nodules beneath the surface of the legs' skin. A loofah or brush should be used on dry legs and applied in long, sweeping, upward motions—from foot to knee, then knee to groin. After using the loofah, bathe and apply a moisturizing cream or lotion.

If you have a red rash that looks like permanent goose bumps, it may be due to lack of Vitamin A in your diet, and will not respond to topical applications.

Knees are often the driest part of the leg; special attention with moisturizers or the loofah should alleviate the problem. On some people, however, the skin on the knees is not only dry but dark and coarse as well. You can lighten darkened knees with commercial skin-lighteners, or you can bleach the skin yourself with a mixture of salt and lemon juice. Remember to moisturize after either treatment.

◆ TAKING IT OFF

There are three methods of hair removal: shaving, using a depilatory, and waxing.

Shaving is the simplest way of removing hair, but it must be done frequently and does not leave your skin especially smooth. There is nothing you can do about the speed at which your leg hair grows back after shaving, but you can minimize the roughening effects of shaving.

Be sure to soften the skin first, either with soap and water or with shaving lather. Allow the softening agent to work for a few moments, then slowly draw the razor against your legs in the *same* direction as the hair grows. Don't soften your legs with any creams or lotions that will gum up the razor.

Depilatories leave your skin smoother than shaving and need to be applied only about twice a month. A depilatory works by penetrating your skin and dissolving the hair. To accomplish this, the depilatory must contain strong chemicals, which have a drying effect on your legs. So be sure to choose a reputable brand; don't try to save money on a depilatory. Apply a moisturizing lotion or cream to your legs after using any depilatory.

Waxing produces the smoothest legs of all. There are two types of waxing—hot and cold. Cold waxing can be done at home with kits available at drugstores and cosmetics counters. If you choose hot waxing, I recommend that you have it done professionally. By doing it yourself, you run the risk of burning your skin. Hot waxing works by spreading wax on the skin, letting it cool, and then pulling it off. Pulling off the wax also pull the hairs out by the roots. There is some pain involved, and you have to let your leg hair grow to at least 1/4 inch before wax can be applied.

An alternative to hair removal is bleaching. Although there are several ammonia/peroxide products available for home use, I recommend that you have the job done professionally. Amateur application of bleaches can lead to skin irritation or an allergic reaction—or result in exotic hair color you weren't expecting.

No matter how you remove (or bleach) your leg hair, watch for side effects. If you have any irritation, allergic reaction, or infection, switch to another method. If the symptom persists for more than a few days, consult a dermatologist.

◆ TO TAN OR NOT TO TAN

Tan legs may look healthier than pale legs, but are they? Certainly anyone returning to a winter climate after a spell at the beach will look healthier than someone who has been left behind to battle snow, sleet, and slush. But how much of that healthy look is due to tanning and how much due to a period of relaxation away from everyday cares and concerns? A tan is only a by-product of a vacation; the true health benefits come from the rest and relaxation.

In our culture, a tan is often associated with success and sex appeal, so those who can't get away to the "real thing" sometimes go to great lengths to look as though they've just stepped off the beach or the ski slopes. There are self-tanning lotions and gels, tan accelerators, tanning pills, solar lamps, and tanning parlors. Not all of these methods are equally effective—or equally benign.

Personally, I think lightly tanned legs are more attractive

than pale legs, but there are sensible and not-so-sensible ways of getting a tan.

Tanning is a normal reaction to the sun's rays; it is a defense mechanism of the skin against the aggression of the sun. However, a sunburn is a sign that ultraviolet rays have penetrated the outer skin and reached the skin's deeper layers. There, the ultraviolet rays traumatize the cells, blood vessels, and connective tissue. Inflammation appears on the surface of the skin.

Years may pass before you notice the skin damage caused by too much exposure to the sun. Your skin may age prematurely, become blotchy and wrinkled, or develop skin cancer. These complications are related to the total amount of ultraviolet rays you have been exposed to over the years.

So how can you avoid the potential dangers of sun exposure, short of avoiding the sun completely or covering your entire body with clothing? Luckily, a wide range of excellent sunscreens and sun blocks is readily available today. These products either absorb or reflect the sun's damaging rays, thereby protecting your skin.

The label of any sunscreen will tell you its SPF—sun protection factor. A sunscreen with an SPF of 4 will allow you to stay in the sun without burning 4 times longer than you could stay if you wore no sunscreen. For example, if you normally burn after one hour in the sun, an application of SPF 4 sunscreen will allow you to stay in the sun for four hours without burning. The highest SPF generally available is 15; a few less widely available preparations have an SPF of 25 or even higher.

Sun blocks are composed of chemical agents that reflect the sun's rays. They offer total protection from the sun; you will not burn, but you will not tan either. Be sure to reapply any sunscreen or block after swimming or exercise. Unlike skin lotions, sunscreens must be of good quality. Don't go for the cheapest product. Buy one with a good reputation.

"Sun tan" lotions, oils, or gels that do not display an SPF offer no protection from the sun. Most are made with a base of mineral or coconut oils. They lubricate the skin but do not promote tanning, despite their claims. Use these products only if you tan very easily and require no protection from the sun. All others should use a sunscreen lotion with an SPF.

Now let's take a closer look at artificial tanning methods. I recommend that you stay well away from tanning pills, which contain hazardous dyes. Solar lamps are dangerous, too, because they cause premature aging and chronic skin damage.

Because there are so many tanning parlors around today—some calling themselves clinics or institutes and purporting to promote good health—I feel I must discuss them at some length.

Tanning parlors replace the sun with lamps that give off more burning rays than the sun does; one-half hour in a tanning parlor exposes you to three to ten times more burning rays than the same time spent with unprotected skin under a midday tropical sun.

Tanning parlor promoters often claim that the exposure they give you prepares your skin to receive the types of rays that tan you. This is false.

The promoters also claim that their treatments have a "therapeutic" effect on your skin and your health. False again. The strong rays in tanning parlors can actually induce inflammation and connective-tissue damage in and around your blood vessels. Exposure at tanning parlor levels can damage the lens of your eye and lead to cataracts.

I recommend only two artificial tanning products—self-tanning lotions and gels, and tan accelerators. Self-tanning products give you color without any sun exposure and wash off gradually a few days after application. Tan accelerators promote faster tanning when you do go out into the sun. They are applied once a day at least three days prior to exposure.

TLC works. You need not expose your legs to harmful products or methods in your quest for smooth, moist, lightly tanned legs. As you know, TLC can make your Great Legs more attractive and healthier, too—quickly and easily.

8

A GLIMPSE OF STOCKING

What to wear to flatter and show off your Great Legs.

High-rise hemlines may be the rage of the runways, but your common sense will tell you if short skirts are for you. Even if you have achieved your Great Legs (and they are as healthy, strong, and smooth as possible), heredity, age, and lifestyle may not be in your favor where short skirts are concerned.

Besides, there is much more than mere hem length to consider when choosing fashions for your Great Legs. There is garment shape and cut, fabric texture and pattern, shoe type, heel height, color coordination.

To find hide-and-chic solutions for your fashion problems, I consulted Adele Smith, one of Florida's foremost fashion experts. A down-to-earth sort, she is in favor of dressing to suit yourself: "Don't follow fashion out the window," Adele advises. "Always wear what's most flattering for *you*. If you're a heavy-set woman, you know better than to wear a red satin minidress."

If you are among the lucky few for whom thigh-high skirts are appropriate, Adele offers these suggestions. The uniformity of a coordinated look—opaque stockings that match your miniskirt—will make you look taller. Contrasting hose will make you look shorter. She warns, however, that coordination can get out of hand. "If you're wearing a yellow minidress, putting on yellow stockings is going to make you look more like a chicken than anything else." So take care to vary shade or texture when putting together a coordinated look.

In general, Adele advises to keep an eye on fabric textures and proportions when dressing to disguise leg problems. A bulky fabric will produce a bulky look. A large pattern will make you look large; a busy one will attract attention. Vertical lines, in garment construction and in fabrics, create the illusion of height.

Comfort and fit are also important for dressing to your legs' best advantage. Tight, restrictive clothing is not good for your circulation. You cannot feel comfortable and at ease in clothes that are too tight, or that do not fit well for any other reason. No matter how much you like a garment—even if it is one recommended for your particular case—do not buy it if it does not fit perfectly.

If you are dressing to disguise heavy legs, remember that "less is more." The less cluttered your clothes are, the smoother you will look. Wear whatever colors are flattering to you, but avoid bright colors at problem areas; they will only draw attention to the very feature you are trying to disguise.

If your problem is too-thin legs, compensate for your lack of curves with "curves" in your clothes. Use gathers, pleats, tucks, and ruffles to offset your straight planes and angles.

Here are some suggestions for solving specific fashion problems.

◆ IF YOUR LEGS ARE TOO HEAVY

DO WEAR:
- A-line skirts with medium-full bottoms that end 1 or 2 inches below the knee at the slimmest part of your calf
- Straight-leg slacks without pleats or gathers
- Garments and fabrics with vertical lines
- Medium-to-dark stockings
- Stockings and shoes in tones that blend with lower garment color.
- Shoes with an open toe or open heel.

AVOID WEARING:
- Short skirts or short shorts
- Gathered skirts
- Tight slacks
- Light- or bright-colored stockings
- Delicate shoes

◆ IF YOUR THIGHS ARE TOO HEAVY

DO WEAR:
- Loose fitting, slightly flared skirts and dresses that end 1 or 2 inches below the knee at the slimmest part of your calf
- Full-cut slacks

- Culottes or roomy walking shorts
- A skirted bathing suit or one with "shorts-type" legs
- Darker colors on the bottom than on the top
- Vertical lines in fabric and garment design
- Medium to lightweight fabrics

AVOID WEARING:

- Pleated skirts or slacks
- Anything that draws attention to the thigh area: patch pockets on thighs or derrière, fancy zippers, rhinestones, studding, and so on
- Short skirts or short shorts
- Clingy skirts, slacks, or shorts
- Tight jeans
- Any garment or belt that cinches your waist
- A maillot bathing suit or one with high-cut legs
- A light-color bottom garment with a darker top garment
- Bulky or heavily textured fabrics

◆ IF YOUR ANKLES ARE TOO THICK

DO WEAR:

- Slacks, if the problem is severe
- Medium-to-dark stockings
- Pumps or sling-back shoes with 1-inch heels

AVOID WEARING:

- Long dresses and slacks that end just above the ankle
- Light-colored stockings, shoes, and boots
- Delicate or flat-heeled shoes; shoes with straps at the instep; shoes that are cut low on the sides
- Bright-colored or intricately-patterned stockings

◆ IF YOUR LEGS ARE TOO THIN

DO WEAR:

- Pleated or gathered skirts and dresses with hems just below the knee
- Pleated slacks in medium to heavyweight fabrics

- Garments and fabrics with horizontal lines
- Neutral-tone stockings
- Simple, delicate shoes; strappy sandals; low-cut pumps

AVOID WEARING:
- A-line skirts and dresses
- Short skirts
- Tight skirts and slacks
- Solid, dark colors
- Dark-colored stockings
- Heavy, chunky shoes

◆ IF YOUR LEGS ARE SHORT

DO WEAR:
- Bathing suits that are cut high on the leg
- Skirt and dress hems at the top of your calf
- Slacks with clean, vertical lines
- Shoes and stockings that are toned to your skirt, dress, or slacks to create the longest possible line from waist to toes
- Shoes with a low and narrow or V-shaped vamp

AVOID WEARING:
- Skirts or dresses with patterns or decorations at the hem
- Slacks with cuffs
- Any garment that cuts the leg in pieces: shorts, bobby sox, knee socks
- Baggy slacks
- Shoes with ankle straps or T-straps

◆ PROBLEM FEET

To make **wide, short feet** seem longer and narrower, wear:
- Shoes that taper to a pointed, not rounded toe
- Sandals with angled straps that wrap over the instep

To make **long, narrow feet** seem shorter and wider wear:
- Shoes with wide straps
- Sandals with wide, straight straps

Choosing clothes for your Great Legs will be easier if you follow these guidelines, but the most important thing to consider is how the clothes make you feel. If you are dressing to please someone else or because fashion dictates you should dress a certain way, then you will not feel or look your best. If, however, you feel attractive and comfortable in your clothes, then they are the right ones for *you*.

9

IN A SERIOUS VEIN

Why you get varicose veins; what you can do to prevent and treat them.

◆ HOW IT ALL BEGINS...

t all started with my second pregnancy, Dr. Lanctôt."
"My new job keeps me on my feet all day."
"It must be because I put on a lot of weight."
Many patients who consult me because of their varicose veins are convinced they know what started the problem. And as far as they go, my patients' observations are correct. Pregnancy, a job that keeps you standing (or sitting) all day, and weight gain *are* serious aggravating factors in the evolution of vein disease.

On their own, however, these factors won't produce sick veins. It takes a predisposition for varicose veins to develop.

Varicose veins are an inherited disease.

Most patients are surprised when I ask them about the condition of both their mothers' and their fathers' veins. Contrary to popular belief, men *are* affected by varicose veins, and to the same extent as women where the large saphenous veins are concerned. Men, however, rarely suffer from the tiny spider viens that so often affect women.

Before we go any further, let's talk about exactly what varicose veins are. Simply put, they are veins that are dilated and unable to carry blood back to the heart. The blood either stagnates in the veins or flows in the wrong direction entirely. The valves that regulate the blood flow in the veins may be working improperly or may have stopped working altogether.

Varicose veins have different names according to the size of the vein involved.

Spider veins, often called broken capillaries, are the small, bluish varicose veins most often found on the sides and back parts of the legs. They usually appear before the larger veins have become varicose. Spider veins, while relatively harmless, are often unsightly enough to discourage wearing bathing suits and shorts. The **reticular**, or middle-sized, **veins** of the superficial system also become varicose, but they are not as visible as spider veins.

The most serious varicose problems are found in the **long saphenous vein**, the largest vein in the superficial system.

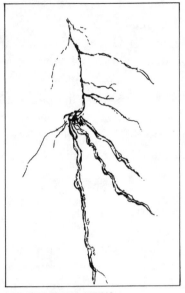

MEDIUM-SMALL VEINS

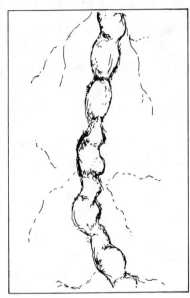

LARGE VEINS

This is the vein on the inside of the leg that becomes visibly enlarged, knotted, or swollen by deterioration. The **short saphenous vein,** which ends behind the knee and after traveling up from the outside of the lower leg, is sometimes affected as well, although much less frequently than the long saphenous vein. Problems in the saphenous veins are especially serious because they affect the other veins that drain into them.

Although heredity is the major cause of varicose veins, there are other ways in which the protective valves in your veins may be damaged. These are thrombophlebitis, trauma, and, in rare instances, particularly strenuous physical effort.

Thrombophlebitis is an inflammation caused by a blood clot in the deep veins of your calf, thigh, or pelvis. This clotting can occur after surgery, after childbirth, or without any apparent reason. While the blood clot itself will clear up in six to eighteen months, the valves in the veins may be so damaged that they can no longer prevent the blood from flowing downward. A high-pressure system builds up that eventually works it way to the surface veins, which then dilate and become varicose.

Trauma—any accident or injury to the leg—can also damage the valves in the legs. And as I've said, damaged valves can lead to vein dilation and varicose veins. Only in very rare instances, however, does strenuous physical effort lead to varicose veins, but it can and does occur. Lifting a very heavy object or pushing against a strong opposing force can so increase the pressure in your veins that a valve explodes. The related veins will then dilate and become varicose.

I have already cited pregnancy, long periods of sitting or standing, weight gain, and aging as aggravating factors in the development of varicose veins. These factors will not cause varicose veins; but, if you have an inherited predisposition, they will increase the likelihood of your developing varicose veins. Other aggravating factors are: heat, alcohol and spices, tight clothing, chronic constipation, prolonged bed rest, and unsuitable shoes.

Varicose veins develop during pregnancy because of increased pressure on the veins caused by the expanding womb; increased volume of blood flowing through the veins; and an increased level of sex hormones in the blood, which is thought to relax the muscle tissue in the walls of the veins, thus causing distension and varicosity. Many women find that their varicose veins become more prominent and uncomfortable during pregnancy. Others find that they suddenly start to develop spider veins and other small varicose veins. But no major veins will become varicose without hereditary predisposition, regardless of how many pregnancies you have. Delivery brings relief to those women whose existing varicose veins have been aggravated by pregnancy. In women who have developed varicose veins during pregnancy the varicose veins often disappear after the birth. Any varicose vein that is left two months after delivery will remain permanently.

Any job that requires long hours of physical restriction—either standing or sitting— greatly increases the risk of developing varicose veins. Immobility reduces the muscular pump activity in your legs, which causes the blood to stagnate in the veins. Eventually, the veins become dilated and varicose. Prolonged bed rest affects veins the same way.

Being overweight is one of the most common aggravating factors associated with varicose veins, especially if you are more than 20 percent over your ideal weight. The added weight you carry puts an extra burden on your veins. The veins have to fight the increased pressure caused by excess weight.

Aging brings not only a decrease in physical activity but a decrease in the amount of muscle in the body. As a result, the muscular pumping of the legs becomes less effective and returns blood to the heart less efficiently. Again, this causes the stagnation and dilation that aggravates an inherited tendency to varicose veins.

Heat can cause varicose veins to swell and become uncomfortable. It can also create new varicose veins by causing veins to dilate. Heat comes from many sources: climate; living or working environment; hot baths; tight, warm boots; excessive sunbathing; or even frequent leg-waxing.

Alcohol and spices also cause veins to dilate, as does tight clothing that impedes the return of blood to your heart. Along with tight boots, girdles, garters, and knee-high stockings (other than the kind made especially to compress the leg) are the worst offenders.

Chronic constipation also aggravates the tendency toward varicose veins. A bowel loaded with stool compresses the large veins in your pelvic area, causing increased blood drainage into your legs. Straining to evacuate the bowel increases the pressure on the veins in your abdominal cavity. This added pressure will also be passed on to the veins in your legs.

Finally, unsuitable shoes are an aggravating factor. Wearing shoes without heels (such as ballet slippers) leads to flat feet. Flat feet prevent the venous pump in your foot from working. Shoes with heels that are too high can also keep the pump from working properly. Ideally, you should walk barefooted as much as possible—on the beach if you are geographically fortunate, in your home in any case. And you should always select shoes with good support and sensible heels.

For women without varicose veins that means 1-inch heels for working, higher heels for occasional evening wear, and comfortable commonsense shoes—such as good walking shoes, sturdy sandals, or crepe-soled lace-up shoes—the rest of the time.

◆ SO WHAT CAN I DO?

For women with varicose veins these same recommendations about shoes apply. In addition, you must wear support stockings and—*this is mandatory*—walk at least one mile each day. Exercising and wearing support, or compression, stockings are the main things you can do to prevent varicose veins if you have inherited the tendency to develop them. (After all, it's too late to change your parents!)

Most of my patients groan when I suggest wearing support hose. "They're horrible," they complain. "My mother had to wear them. They're thick, ugly, and uncomfortable."

Well, let me reassure you—the hosiery industry has changed a few things since your mother's day. Today, support stockings are lightweight, supple, elegant, and comfortable; and they come in a variety of fashionable colors, textures, and styles.

This new generation of support hose also comes in the form of knee-high stockings. But do not confuse regular knee-high stockings with compression ones.

In compression stockings (knee-high or full-length) the pressure is greatest at the ankle; compression decreases as the stocking moves up the leg. This helps the blood return to the upper portion of the leg and from there to the heart. Regular knee-high stockings, on the other hand, block circulation with their band of pressure in the middle of the leg; they are an obstacle to venous blood flow and can worsen a varicose condition.

Control-top pantyhose, by compressing and restricting blood flow in the upper thigh and groin area where the junction of the long saphenous vein and the deep vein system lies, can also aggravate a varicose condition.

We've already talked about the benefits of exercise on your

Great Legs, but let's look at exercise again in the context of varicose veins.

If you have varicose veins, the circulation in your legs has been curtailed; there are less fully-functioning veins to return the blood to the heart. Exercising slows down the spread of the condition by strengthening and enlarging the leg muscles. The larger those muscles are, the more pressure they can exert on your deep veins. The flow of blood back to your heart through the deep veins creates a negative pressure, rather like a vacuum effect, on the superficial veins. The stronger that pressure, the better the drainage in your superficial veins. Blood will not stagnate and dilate the superficial veins, and they will less likely become varicose.

Exercise is also important for increasing respiration. Breathing has a similar suction effect on the veins; the deeper you breathe, the greater the vacuum effect on your veins. That is, more blood is sucked back up to the heart.

Remember also that blood must flow against the force of gravity to return to the heart. By increasing muscle strength and respiration, exercise also helps to overcome the effects of gravity.

You can get gravity to work *with* you in returning the blood to your heart by elevating your legs above your head. Such a position speeds up the circulation rate of stagnating venous blood, which then returns to the heart with the help of gravity. Here are two exercises. Either one, done once a day, will give your legs the benefit of gravity for a change.

1. Lie on the floor, keeping your back flat against the floor and your derrière about three inches from the wall. Rest your feet against the wall. Hold this position for as long as it is comfortable.

2. Lie on your back [Diagram A] with your legs extended in front of you and your arms at your sides. Lift your legs, making sure to keep the small of the back on the floor, so that they are at a right angle to your body. (If the small of your back is not flat against the floor, bend your knees until it is.) Raise your buttocks from the floor, supporting the small of your back with your

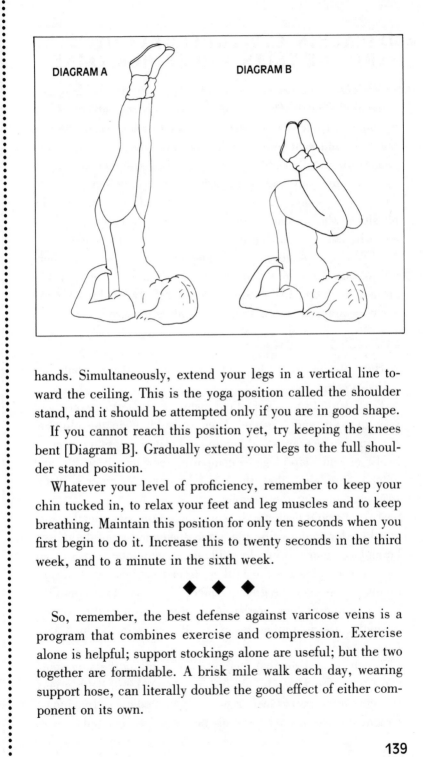

hands. Simultaneously, extend your legs in a vertical line toward the ceiling. This is the yoga position called the shoulder stand, and it should be attempted only if you are in good shape.

If you cannot reach this position yet, try keeping the knees bent [Diagram B]. Gradually extend your legs to the full shoulder stand position.

Whatever your level of proficiency, remember to keep your chin tucked in, to relax your feet and leg muscles and to keep breathing. Maintain this position for only ten seconds when you first begin to do it. Increase this to twenty seconds in the third week, and to a minute in the sixth week.

So, remember, the best defense against varicose veins is a program that combines exercise and compression. Exercise alone is helpful; support stockings alone are useful; but the two together are formidable. A brisk mile walk each day, wearing support hose, can literally double the good effect of either component on its own.

◆ DIAGNOSIS AND TREATMENT OF VARICOSE VEINS AND SPIDER VEINS

Varicose veins never occur before puberty unless there is a congenital defect. Their onset occurs with the advent of sex hormones. Their development is related to hormonal changes that take place at puberty, during pregnancy, and at menopause. Untreated, varicose veins will always worsen with age.

If you are concerned about varicose veins or spider veins and decide to seek medical advice, I recommend that you consult a physician who specializes in the treatment of vein disease. Doctors who lack experience in this field may, unfortunately, dismiss your complaint as trivial and may discourage treatment unless your veins are visibly and seriously affected. A vein specialist, however, will evaluate you carefully, looking for the early warning signs that signal impending disease.

DIAGNOSIS

Here is what would happen if you consulted me about your varicose veins.

First, I would take a medical history and question you about your heredity and lifestyle. Then I would begin the physical examination. As you stood before me I would assess the general health of your (bare) legs by comparing their length, width, and color (one against the other) and by checking your skin for swelling, inflammation, or ulcers.

Next, I would evaluate the condition of the superficial veins, checking for spider veins and noting the condition of the reticular and saphenous veins. I would also examine the veins in your feet. These veins are the farthest from your heart and, accordingly, experience the greatest effect of gravity. They contain a wealth of information. Spider veins on the inside of the foot, for example, are an indication of insufficiency in the long saphenous vein.

Touch is my principal method for examining the superficial venous system. I may be old-fashioned, but I still believe very strongly in the importance of touching in medicine. Touching a patient informs me not only about the veins, but tells me as well about the texture of the skin, the strength and tension of the muscles, and so forth. It also puts me "in touch" with the energy and spirit of my patient. The more I touch a patient, the better I am at treating her, and the sooner I get excellent results.

The most important vein to examine by touch is the long saphenous vein. When deterioration is so advanced as to be visible, diagnosing saphenous vein insufficiency is not at all difficult—the vein is tortuously knotted and swollen. In the past, because doctors lacked the treatment options available today, the accepted practice was to let the long saphenous vein deteriorate until your child bearing years were over. Now we believe that the sooner you get treatment, the less trouble you'll have in the long run.

It is, however, difficult to make an early diagnosis of insufficiency of the long saphenous vein. For this reason I have developed a special set of criteria that I, and all the doctors in my clinics, use to spot insufficiency as soon as the long saphenous vein begins to become incompetent.

The only exception to this rule of touching to examine the superficial vein system is when there is difficulty in locating the junction of the short saphenous vein. Because this junction controls the connection between the superficial and deep vein systems, it is important to locate it precisely. If the junction is not where it is assumed to be and I cannot palpate, or feel, it superficially, then I may order a special X ray, known as a varicogram, before I begin treatment.

Examining and diagnosing the deep vein system is very different from examining and diagnosing the superficial vein system. Touch does not work on the deep veins because they are buried beneath muscles where we can neither see nor palpate them. But certain clues, like reddening or port-wine stains on the skin, legs of different lengths, or swelling can suggest the possibility of disease in the deep vein system. If such indications are present, I will arrange for one of several tests. These include: ultrasound (showing the direction of the flow of blood), venogram (a special X ray that shows the veins), or plethysmography (a measure of venous pressure).

Once I have examined and evaluated your superficial vein system and ruled out disease in the deep vein system, I can tell you how your particular case of varicose veins will develop. Of course, I will also have taken your medical history, heredity, and lifestyle into account for this prognosis. Then, I would recommend a course of treatment.

TREATMENT

There are three forms of treatment for varicose veins: sclerotherapy (injection therapy), surgery, and compression therapy.

Sclerotherapy

The most commonly used treatment is sclerotherapy, in which the affected veins are injected with a medical substance known as a sclerosing agent. The timely introduction of this treatment can arrest the progress of the diseased veins.

Sclerotherapy injections induce a healing process in which the treated veins thicken and close up. This creates scar tissue under the skin, turning the veins into hard cords. These cords subside in about a month, leaving no trace of either the treatment or the veins. Spider veins disappear in one week. The discomfort and unsightliness caused by the affected veins disappear as well. Since the veins that are treated have ceased to function properly, the blood has already been rerouted through other veins. Closing off the affected veins with injection therapy can only improve your circulation. The blood is no longer "fooled" into trying to enter nonfunctioning veins and takes a better, more direct route back to the heart.

Which veins can be treated? Every varicose vein or spider vein, whatever its size, can be treated successfully with injections. The saphenous vein itself also responds to sclerotherapy, but there is a high recurrence of varicosity in saphenous veins treated with injections. This high rate of recurrence often makes surgery the preferred treatment for varicose saphenous veins.

When should veins be treated? As we've said, the sooner the better. Left untreated, existing varicose veins become more dilated, affecting connecting veins and forming new varicose veins.

What is the treatment like? First, your physician will mark the exact location of the sick veins. While you're standing, he or she will trace with a pen the general distribution of the varicose veins in your leg.

For the treatment itself—which takes place entirely in the doctor's office—you'll lie down on an examining table, where the doctor will administer the injections. The number of injections can vary from one to forty per session, but about twenty is average. The needles used are very fine, of an almost hairlike thinness, so there is no pain involved; each injection produces only a sensation similar to a pinprick.

Every point of injection will be covered with a cotton ball and tape. Your doctor will instruct you to remove the cotton and tape about two hours after the treatment, while you are soaking in a bath to which baby oil or mineral oil has been added.

Treatments last about fifteen minutes. Depending on the severity of your case, a course of treatment usually takes from one to fifteen weekly sessions. However, the average treatment is eight sessions.

During the course of the treatment you are free to go about your normal activities, including work. Many of my patients receive their treatments during their lunch hours or coffee breaks. You may walk and exercise as much as you like. In fact, you are encouraged to do so.

The only thing to avoid, and then only for the first two days after treatment, is sunbathing. Tape makes the skin more sensitive to the sun, and a brown pigmentation may result (although this is not permanent and will fade in time). If you must go out in the sun during this period, apply a sunscreen with a sun-protection factor of at least 15.

What are the results of sclerotherapy? When injection therapy is done well, the results can be spectacular. Patients often cannot believe the degree of improvement. In cases where the disease was particularly advanced, legs can literally "change" color. For many, the results mean being able to live fully again for the first time in years. Without the discomfort and embarrassment of bulging or discolored veins, they can wear bathing suits and shorts, swim, play tennis, do anything they want.

The veins that are treated have been closed off and cannot come back after treatment. The treatment cannot, however, alter your heredity. You will still have the tendency to form new varicose veins.

So it's important to exercise, wear support hose, and visit your doctor every six months to get the most out of your injection therapy.

Are there any complications or side effects from sclerotherapy? Serious complications resulting from injection therapy are very rare. Still, it is important to acknowledge that there may be some complications.

An allergic reaction to the sclerosing agent is one possibility. This could result in a slight tingling sensation and/or red blotches on the skin. These reactions disappear rapidly, in a matter of minutes or hours. In very rare cases, the allergic reaction could be so severe as to send a patient into shock.

Cases of thrombophlebitis and pulmonary embolism have been reported in past medical literature, but these are extremely rare. Over 60,000 patients have been treated in my clinics, and we've never had any of these problems occur.

If the sclerosing agent is accidentally injected into the subcutaneous tissue or into an arteriole (a small artery), an ulcer may develop. Depending on its size, the ulcer will heal in a few weeks or months; and it will leave a small scar.

Side effects are not uncommon, but they are not serious.

Bruises can appear during the treatment; they will disappear within two to three weeks.

When many small varicose veins are injected, tiny red spots

may appear. These will disappear within three weeks.

Occasionally, tiny red cords will appear in the treated veins. They are caused by a slight inflammation. Walking, compression, and cool, soothing compresses easily cure any such inflammation.

In rare instances, the skin near the site of the injections darkens due to a sensitivity to or too much of the sclerosing agent. Usually the stain will fade and the skin will regain its normal pigmentation.

Occasionally, small spider veins may appear as a side effect of injecting and closing off larger veins. These spider veins, however, are easily treated by further injections.

Other questions I am frequently asked about sclerotherapy:

Q. Have I waited too long to benefit from this treatment?

A. No. It is always better to treat varicose veins than to ignore them. Something can always be done. The treatment may take longer, but the results can be as good.

Q. Am I too old for these treatments?

A. No. Age is no deterrent if you are in good health. I have a patient who first came for treatment when she was 79. She's well into her 80s now; she and her veins are doing just fine.

Q. When is injection therapy not advisable?

A. Sclerotherapy is not advisable if you have any of the following medical conditions: arterial insufficiency; recent thrombophlebitis; an acute infection; or any serious illness. You also should not have injection therapy while you are pregnant.

Q. Will I have to wear bandages after treatment?

A. No, because the top-to-bottom method of sclerotherapy that we use requires no bandaging.

What should I know about choosing a doctor? The success of your treatments will depend on the skill of the doctor you choose. Here are some criteria for evaluating a physician's qualifications to perform sclerotherapy:

- Training. Deal only with a licensed physician. Ask the doctor where he or she trained and how long the training lasted. At a minimum, the doctor should have undergone a month of full-time phlebology training.
- Experience. Ask the doctor how long he or she has been practicing and how many patients he or she has treated. Doctors, like everyone else, develop skill with practice.
- Specialization. Find out where the emphasis lies in the doctor's practice. Does the doctor perform sclerotherapy as only a small part of his or her regular practice, or is it the doctor's principal medical activity?
- Precision. The doctor should be able to tell you, on your first visit, exactly what your diagnosis is, what your prognosis is, and how many treatments you will need. And finally, remember that it is *always* a good idea to get a second opinion—and compare fees.

Surgery

Only the long or short saphenous vein, when varicose, is a candidate for surgical removal, called stripping. The procedure of removal of the long saphenous vein can be performed in one of two ways—long stripping or short stripping. We have been performing short-stripping on the long saphenous vein for the past ten years, and definitely prefer it to long-stripping. Here are the two basic procedures:

Long-Stripping. This operation removes the entire long saphenous vein. It is usually performed in conjunction with a procedure called segmental ligation, which ties off the branch veins leading to the long saphenous vein.

Long-stripping and segmental ligation is a major surgical procedure. The operation, which lasts three hours, is performed under general anesthesia, and it requires a hospital stay of three to five days. It involves a convalescence period of one or two months. It also leaves the patient with ten to twenty scars on each leg, depending on the number of segmental ligations that were necessary.

Short-Stripping. When sclerotherapy is available, it is possible to remove only the upper portion (knee to groin) of the long saphenous vein. The closing off of branch veins can be accomplished with injection only. Because short-stripping does not touch any of the saphenous vein's branches, it leaves only two scars per leg. They will gradually become unnoticeable.

Short-stripping is performed in the hospital under local anesthesia. First, the saphenous vein is tied-off and cut at two points—one in the groin area (where the saphenous vein connects with the deep vein system) and the other just below the knee. Next, an instrument called a stripper is used to remove the tied-off portion of the vein. If the vein is so severely gnarled or distorted as to prevent stripping in one clean motion, the surgeon will need to make one or two additional incisions.

The operation takes about thirty minutes to perform. The patient returns home the same day, and the recovery period is three days to two weeks.

Some of the advantages of short-stripping are obvious—outpatient surgery, local anesthesia, quicker recovery, less scarring, lower costs.

But the main advantage is a medical one. Short-stripping saves the lower part of the long saphenous vein, thus making it available, *if* it is healthy, in case you ever need heart bypass surgery.

When should surgery be performed? In the past, when surgery was the only method of treating varicose veins, doctors preferred to wait until the disease was well-developed before operating. They reasoned that waiting would prevent repeat surgery on the branches of the long saphenous veins. Female patients were usually advised to postpone vein surgery until their childbearing years were over.

The development of injection therapy has changed all that.

Now that branch veins can be treated with sclerotherapy, doctors recommend operating as soon as it becomes necessary. This is good news for women of childbearing age with saphenous vein problems. If you become pregnant after vein removal, the pregnancy will not aggravate an already painful condition. Any new varicosities that develop during or between pregnancies can easily be treated with sclerotherapy.

What are the results of surgery? Varicose veins that have been removed cannot recur. As is the case with sclerotherapy, however, new varicose veins can form after surgery. It is a little like dental work. When you have a cavity filled, there's no guarantee that new cavities won't form later on.

New varicose veins that form after surgery can't be avoided, since neither surgery nor sclerotherapy can cure a hereditary tendency toward varicose veins. But any new varicose veins that form can be controlled by injection therapy. Exercising and wearing support hose after surgery will discourage the formation of new veins.

Other Surgical Techniques

There are other, less common, operations for treating varicose veins.

One is called a phlebectomy. This procedure involves the removal of varicose veins through many small incisions. It is more commonly performed in Europe than in North America. Advocates of this procedure argue that the small scars that result from this operation are aesthetically superior to the dark pigmentation that sometimes results from sclerotherapy. In my experience, injections rarely result in skin discoloration, and I believe they are preferable to phlebectomy.

Another is vein transplantation. This type of treatment is still very much in the experimental stage. Attempts are being made to replace damaged veins with healthy ones taken from the patient's own body or with artificial veins.

Compression Therapy

If poor health or other factors mentioned previously rule out sclerotherapy or surgery, varicose veins can still be treated with compression therapy.

In this method elastic bandages or stockings are used to compress surface veins to help them do what they have lost the power to do on their own.

Compression can help you live with your varicose veins, but it is not a cure. I call it the "aspirin" of varicose vein treatment; it is an excellent palliative for relieving pain and swelling and for preventing further deterioration. Compression therapy is more effective when it is combined with as much physical activity as the patient's health can tolerate.

When are elastic bandages used? Elastic bandages are reserved for the more acute stages of varicose vein disease, when severe complications have set in. Your doctor, of course, will be the one to assess the seriousness of your condition and tell you if bandages are needed and for how long you are likely to have to wear them. The doctor will also select the correct degree of elasticity for your condition. He or she will put the bandages on for you and teach you how to wrap them yourself and instruct you in their care.

A special type of elastic bandage, called the Unna Paste boot, is used to treat a varicose ulcer, which is a wound that develops because of poor skin nutrition. It is simply an elastic bandage coated with zinc. After it has been applied, it dries on the leg in the shape of a boot. It is changed weekly until the ulcer heals.

When are elastic stockings used? Once the acute phase of your vein problem has been alleviated by an elastic bandage, you will be able to maintain the treatment by wearing elastic stockings. Like elastic bandages, elastic stockings vary in their degree of elasticity. They are graded according to the amount of pressure they exert on the leg. The greater the compression, the thicker the stocking.

Medium-compression stockings are usually recommended for post-operative swelling, during pregnancy, and after a varicose ulcer has healed.

Strong-compression stockings are usually ordered in cases of postphlebitic syndrome, chronic venous insufficiency, and persistent serious swelling.

Extra-strong compression is required for lymphedema, a condition that results in grossly swollen legs.

Do not confuse elastic stockings with support hose. Support hose are used only for prevention when an underlying tendency to varicose veins exists or in conjunction with exercise as a preventative after surgery or sclerotherapy. Support hose can be purchased in department or drug stores. Elastic stockings are always prescribed by a doctor and must be purchased at a pharmacy or medical/surgical supply outlet. They are not at all sheer and are not attractive.

So, as you can see, varicose veins are not a condition you must "live with." There are effective therapies for everyone. For many women and men, getting rid of varicose veins has changed their lives. You're never too old and it's never too late—or too early—to do something about your varicose veins. All the treatments I've outlined here—exercise and support hose for prevention, sclerotherapy, surgery, and compression therapy—improve circulation. And, as I've said before, good circulation is one of the key factors in achieving your Great Legs.

10

WALKING

FOR

TWO

How

to

keep

your

Great

Legs

during

pregnancy.

Great expectations?

Well, expect your legs to have their own reaction to your pregnancy. After all, you're going to be carrying significantly more weight; there'll be an overabundance of blood and hormones surging through your body, and you'll be considerably less active than you've been in your nonpregnant past.

During pregnancy, particularly the early part of it, varicose veins may appear for the first time, or an existing varicose condition may worsen. There are three reasons for this.

First, as the womb grows to accommodate the fetus, your pelvic veins are subject to increased pressure, which is in turn transmitted to the surface veins of your legs.

Second, your blood volume increases. There is simply more blood for your veins to carry, which can cause them to dilate and become varicose.

Third, the level of sex hormones in your blood rises. Although the process is not yet completely understood, these hormones are thought to relax the muscle tissue in the walls of your veins; this relaxation increases the likelihood of your veins becoming distended and varicose. (The effect of sex hormones on varicose veins is also evident, to a lesser degree, during the menstrual cycle. Many patients report that their veins are swollen and uncomfortable just before their periods.)

For women with a hereditary tendency toward varicose veins, pregnancy is a dangerous time. High-risk women will probably notice varicose veins forming early in pregnancy. Even women without a hereditary tendency may see varicose veins forming. If you are in the high-risk category, watch for these symptoms:

♦ spider veins developing on your thighs
♦ more pain in existing varicose veins and/or new varicosities in surface veins
♦ vulval varicosities

Often, during pregnancy, surface veins near the entrance to the vagina and veins on the upper inner side of the thighs expand and become varicose. These veins can be alarming in appearance and sometimes uncomfortable, but they are not a serious medical problem. They begin to shrink immediately after delivery and often disappear completely.

Venous pain may appear as early as two weeks after conception; to my physician's eye, the symptoms are as significant as a missed period in making an early diagnosis of pregnancy.

Varicose veins that appear for the first time during pregnancy will often disappear after delivery. Even established varicose veins tend to improve then, too. Unfortunately, these same veins are likely to once again become varicose (or more varicose) during your next pregnancy and will become even more prominent during subsequent pregnancies. Unfortunately, they will also tend to disappear less after each subsequent pregnancy.

◆ WHAT YOU CAN DO

Pregnancy need not inevitably damage your venous system. Here are some measures you can take to prevent or alleviate serious symptoms:

EXERCISE.

Brisk walking, bicycling, and swimming are all excellent for your circulation, which is the most important factor in preventing or minimizing varicose veins. Muscle-specific leg exercises will also aid circulation, as well as keeping your legs firm and toned during pregnancy.

Before you begin *any* exercise program during pregnancy, it is critical to get your doctor's approval. Tell your doctor exactly what you propose to do, and get his or her okay for *each specific* exercise.

Remember these points well:
- ◆ Stop exercising immediately if you feel any pain.
- ◆ Exercise at a regular, moderate pace.
- ◆ Control all your movements; don't jerk or jar your body.
- ◆ Stretch slowly and gently.

The American College of Obstetrics and Gynecology advises against doing any exercises while flat on your back after the fourth month of pregnancy. During the first four months of pregnancy your uterus rests, as it normally does, in the pelvic cavity. After the fourth month, the uterus expands vertically into a position where, when lying on your back, it can compress the main blood vessels related to your heart. Such compression can diminish the flow of oxygen to you and your baby.

If your doctor okays them, you need not stop doing the exercises you ordinarily would do on your back, as long as you alter the position in which they are performed. (At the end of this chapter you'll find diagrams and directions for altering the pertinent exercises from Chapter 5.)

WEAR SUPPORT HOSE.

Begin this practice early in your pregnancy. The compression provided by support hose conteracts the dilation of veins and helps return blood to your heart. Put on your support hose first thing in the morning and remove them only when you go to bed. By all means, wear them when you exercise. And as your pregnancy advances, gradually increase the degree of compression your hose supplies. (When you're not pregnant, it's still a good idea to wear support hose before and during your period if your veins give you trouble then.)

AVOID CONSTRICTING GARMENTS.

Any garment—especially underwear—that's too tight will aggravate congestion of the blood in your leg veins.

WEAR SENSIBLE, COMFORTABLE SHOES.

Choose shoes with good support – 1-inch heels for work, good walking or other casual shoes the rest of the time. Avoid high heels and flats.

RESTRICT WEIGHT GAIN.

Of course you will gain weight during pregnancy; you must for your own and your baby's good health. But it is important to keep your weight gain within the limits suggested by your doctor. Excessive weight gain is a serious aggravating factor in varicose veins during pregnancy.

ELEVATE YOUR LEGS WHENEVER POSSIBLE.

Put your feet up regularly throughout the day. While you sleep, raise your feet with pillows. You can also use blocks to raise the lower end of the bed about 12 inches.

By exercising regularly and observing the above precautions, you should be able to maintain strong, healthy legs throughout your pregnancy. Your body will experience great changes during these nine months; your legs will change, too. But following these measures will allow you, after delivery, to more easily regain your pre-pregnancy shape and return to your Great Legs exercise routine.

◆ MUSCLE-SPECIFIC EXERCISES ALTERED FOR PREGNANCY

It is especially important during pregnancy to support your back by holding in the abdominal muscles firmly while exercising. Remember to release your muscles as often as you desire by bending and extending the working leg.

QUADRICEPS EXERCISE #2

Sit on the floor with your left leg bent [Figure 6; p.90]. (You may support your back against a wall.) Lift and lower the right leg, performing an equal number of repetitions with the foot flexed and with the foot pointed. Release the muscle by bending and extending the leg. Switch legs, bending the right and working the left. Don't forget to release the left leg before going on to the next exercise.

OUTER THIGH RELEASE

Do *not* perform this release [Figures 12, 13, 14; p.94]. Instead, lie on your left side, supporting your upper body on your bent left elbow. Bend and draw in your knees so that your thighs are at a right angle to your body. With your right hand clasp your right ankle and gently draw your right leg back. Be careful not to arch your back.

Next, bring the right leg back to the starting position, then extend it toward the ceiling, holding onto the back of your thigh or your calf with your right hand. Repeat this release on the left side after you have worked the left thigh.

INNER THIGH EXERCISE #2 AND INNER THIGH RELEASE

Do *not* perform these two exercises or the release [Figures 16, 17, 18; pp.96, 97]. To release after Inner Thigh Exercise #1, sit up and bring the soles of your feet together. Clasp your left ankle with your left hand, your right ankle with your right hand, and gently press your thighs open with your elbows.

POST-STRETCH SEQUENCE

This may be too difficult for you as your pregnancy advances. Substitute an additional round of the pre-stretch exercises.

11

WHY YOUR LEGS ACHE

And what to do about it.

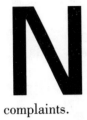 o matter how well you care for your legs, some-
times they hurt—from fatigue, let's say, or per-
haps from too much sitting or standing. There
are many reasons for leg pain, and in this chapter I will examine some of the most common leg
complaints.

◆ GADDING ABOUT

One thing a lot of my patients complain about is travel.
Travel may broaden the mind, but it isn't very kind to the legs.
Long periods of sitting, an inevitable part of travel, interfere
with the return of venous blood to your heart, impairing circulation. Your legs also swell.

There are, however, a number of things you can do to help
your legs weather a long plane or car journey.

- Wear support hose.
- Avoid tight shoes or high, tight boots that will stop your circulation.
- Move around as much as possible. Walk up and down the
aisle on a plane. Stop the car frequently for a short leg stretch
(especially if you are driving and cannot exercise as described below).
- Exercise while sitting. Move your toes inside your shoes.
Flex your feet and rotate your ankles. Stretch your legs out in
front of you and point and flex your feet.
- Do not drink alcoholic beverages on a plane. Alcohol exacer-
bates vein dilation and leg swelling.
- Keep out of the direct path of the car heater. Heat also exac-
erbates vein dilation and leg swelling.

◆ GETTING AN ANGLE ON THE JOB

Anyone looking at a payroll deduction slip can tell you that
work is taxing enough—without having it take a toll on your
legs, too. Again, there are a few simple things you can do to
minimize the impact of long periods of sitting or standing.

If you're desk-bound, try to use a chair that allows for an angle of more than 90 degrees between your upper body and your thighs and legs. The sharp 90-degree angle cuts circulation between the veins in your legs and the venous system leading to the heart. An ideal chair will provide an angle of 120 degrees. An ordinary chair, however, can give you the angle your body needs for good circulation if you elevate its front legs on a thick telephone book.

If you can't change the angle of your chair, you can raise your legs in front of you on a footstool or on a pile of books.

In any case, leave your chair periodically and walk around for a few moments. While sitting, change position as often as possible. Occasionally contract and relax your leg and foot muscles. And don't inhibit your circulation by crossing your legs or ankles. Especially don't tuck your legs under your chair—with your ankles crossed or uncrossed.

If you have to stand on the job, try to move about as much as possible. If you must remain in one place for a long period, try to exercise whenever possible. Here are some unobtrusive movements that will help your circulation. Wriggle your toes inside your shoes. Shift your weight from one foot to the other. Raise your heels, one at a time, an inch or two off the floor. It is also important to wear good support hose that will give your legs adequate compression. And, of course, be sure to wear comfortable shoes that give you good support.

◆ OH, MY ACHING LEGS...

Patients come to me describing all kinds of leg symptoms—heaviness, numbness, tension, swelling, cramps. While most of these symptoms can be traced to causes that are not serious, such sensations are annoying and can adversely affect the quality of your life.

It is sometimes a challenge to pinpoint the cause of such symptoms, but in general there are two categories of causes—venous and nonvenous.

If the problem is in your veins you may experience:

◆ Cramps that wake you at night or that occur as you wake up in the morning.

◆ Numbness when you go to bed. It lasts about thirty minutes to an hour. If you experience this symptom, you may find it easier to fall asleep after someone has massaged your legs.

◆ Leg pain during exercise. Exercise usually relieves venous pain, but sometimes it may aggravate it. Leg pain caused by venous disease is intermittent; you may walk three miles one day without pain, yet experience pain after three blocks the next day. However, this pain rarely forces an abrupt stop in the exercise.

◆ "Restless legs" or the inability to sit still.

◆ Heaviness and aching in the legs after standing for a half-hour or so. This is one of the most common symptoms among people with venous disease.

◆ Leg pain before or during the first days of a menstrual period.

Such pain will be worse in the afternoon and the evening than in the morning. It will be aggravated by long periods of standing or sitting. And it will worsen with heat as well as with physical effort.

Leg pains caused by high pressure in your veins will be aggravated by any increase in vein pressure. Heat, for example, will dilate the vein and increase the volume of blood flowing through it, thereby causing the pressure to go up. Standing in one place for a long time intensifies the pull of gravity on the flow of blood, again increasing pressure and pain. Lifting heavy objects will exert extra pressure on the abdominal veins, which in turn will be passed on to the veins in your legs.

Conversely, any factor that reduces venous hypertension will lessen the pain. Exercise, for example, will activate the muscular pump and force the blood upward. Putting your legs up will lessen the affect of gravity. Wearing compression stockings will prevent veins from dilating.

Leg pains can also be due to nonvenous causes such as:

Arterial disease. If you develop a pain in your calf (or another part of your leg) every time you walk a *specific* distance, say one or two hundred yards, it could be a sign of arteriosclerosis. Such pains are sudden and severe; they force you to interrupt your activity.

Arthritis. Arthritis pain is usually very intense in the morning. Unlike venous pain, leg pain caused by arthritis will also be relieved by the application of heat. Arthritic pain also responds to aspirin and anti-inflammatory drugs unlike venous pain.

Muscular strain. Leg muscles can be hurt by excessive exercise, unfamiliar activity, or any physical stress. If the muscle strain is sudden, that is, not related to chronic wear-and-tear, sports medicine practitioners recommend the RICE treatment: rest, ice, compression, and elevation.

Sciatica. Sciatica is a sharp pain in a body area touched by the sciatic nerve—buttocks, hip, back and outer part of the thigh, the lower leg, ankle, or foot. It is caused by an irritation of the nerve roots that make up the sciatic nerve. Lower back pain frequently accompanies sciatica; lifting a straight leg will worsen the back and leg pain. Rest is the principal treatment, along with analgesics and, at times, physical therapy and special exercises.

Bone bruises, fractures, or tumors. The degree of discomfort from bone pain varies according to its cause. For any pain that seems to emanate from the bone, consult a physician.

There are many causes of leg pain. Some may be serious; most are not. Keep in mind that above all, Great Legs are healthy legs. If you have any uncertainty about any leg symptom you have, consult your physician.

12

More Than Fat, Less Than Lite

How you get cellulite; what you can do to get rid of it.

ellulite (the French pronounce it "celluLEET") is a word coined in the 1920s by French beauticians to describe the dimpled fat deposits found on the hips of even thin women.

Having fat around the hips and thighs is normal for women. Nature's original intention for creating women's capacity to store fat in these areas was an excellent one: infant survival. In a famine, women—particularly those with a greater-than-average tendency to carry fat on their thighs and hips—could go on breastfeeding their babies, thanks to their extra fuel supply.

Cellulite, however, is something more than just fat around the hips and thighs. Even thin women have cellulite—dimpled fat deposits that will not go away no matter how much they diet or exercise. For some reason, the body does not use these fat deposits as a fuel source. If it did, thin women would not have cellulite. There must be some reason why the body does not use cellulite, but it is not yet known.

Cellulite is not only considered unattractive, but is also widely believed to be unhealthy. While most North American health professionals still define cellulite as plain old fat, in many European countries—especially France and Czechoslovakia—doctors believe cellulite to be indicative of impaired venous and lymphatic circulation in the legs and, therefore, a precursor of varicose veins.

◆ WHY YOU DEVELOP CELLULITE

HEREDITY

Some women inherit a tendency to develop cellulite; some do not. While you cannot change your genes, you can minimize the other factors that contribute to cellulite build-up.

SEX HORMONES

There are three ways in which sex hormones, especially estrogen, and cellulite are related. First, the higher your estrogen level, the more likely you are to retain fluid. Fluid is drained from the legs via the lymphatic system, against the pull of gravity. Excess fluid causes the lymph system to bog down, encouraging the formation of cellulite.

Second, estrogen is a female hormone, governing specifically female functions in the body. One of those is to store fat around the hips and thighs. Therefore, the higher your estrogen level, the more likely you are to store fat, some of which the body will not be able to use and which will become cellulite.

Third, fat cells themselves produce estrogen. The larger and more active the fat cells, the more estrogen they produce. This becomes a vicious cycle where cellulite is concerned.

Birth control pills contain significant amounts of estrogen. The longer you've been on the pill, the more likely you are to have cellulite. Going off the pill will not make your cellulite disappear.

Pregnancy also increases estrogen levels, so the more pregnancies you have, the more cellulite you are likely to have. Estrogen levels rise the week before your menstrual period as well. Each year, you are in a high-estrogen state for three months. By the time you reach forty, you've lived through the equivalent of eight premenstrual, high-estrogen years. That certainly helps account for middle-age spread.

DIET

Fatty foods encourage cellulite build-up. Full-fat cheeses, excess animal fat, fried foods, and the coconut, palm, and hydrogenated oils found in so many convenience foods (like artificial dairy products and frosting mixes) should be avoided if you tend to accumulate cellulite.

POOR LYMPH DRAINAGE

Like the vein system, the lymphatic system relies on good pumping action of the muscles to operate efficiently. Forgive the ugly image, but the lymph system is rather like a sewer system that drains off garbage. If you want to lose fat or cellulite from your legs, you must have good lymph drainage. If you have poor lymph drainage in your legs, any fat you lose will be taken from a more accessible region of your body—your throat, breasts, or arms.

The same things that block or impair venous circulation—too little exercise, too much standing, even sitting with your legs crossed—also impair lymph circulation and drainage and encourage the formation of cellulite.

WARPED CONNECTIVE TISSUE

Connective tissue is the thin, fibrous covering that surrounds muscle and acts as a bed for fat cells. When you're young, the tissue is smooth and flat. When you begin to age, the tissue clumps up and warps like a piece of overstretched elastic. Fat then collects in the pockets of warped connective tissue. The warp distorts the texture and consistency of the fat layer, causing the dimples that are characteristic of cellulite.

◆ WHAT YOU CAN DO ABOUT CELLULITE

For many years, when my patients asked me what they could do about cellulite, I answered, "Nothing that I know of can be done." Many were disappointed by my answer, especially the ones who, through successful treatment of varicose veins, had begun to think of their legs as healthy and attractive and wanted to make them even healthier and more attractive. But I knew of no better answer to give.

That was before I met Carola Barczak, nutritionist and massage therapist. In her Figure & Face Salons Ltd. in Toronto and Fort Erie, Ontario, she has treated thousands of women with cellulite problems with a method she developed herself through extensive research. She began her quest for an effective treatment for cellulite when, despite reaching her goal weight, eating well and exercising, she was still unable to get rid of her cellulite.

THE BARCZAK METHOD

Clients at Carola Barczak's salons receive two different treatments. One treatment raises the temperature of the fat in the legs while simultaneously exercising slow-twitch muscles. The other, known as vacusage, encourages lymph drainage. The state of a client's cellulite determines if the first treatment is given alone or if both treatments are given.

In the first treatment, heated pads wrapped around the client's leg raise the temperature of the fat in the leg. This increases the enzyme action of the fat cells, opens circulatory channels and "loosens" cell membranes so that fat can flow out of them. At the same time, a specially designed electro-muscle stimulation machine vigorously exercises the slow-twitch leg muscles by alternately contracting and relaxing the muscles with mild electrical impulses.

In the United States, electro-muscle stimulation (EMS) is usually used by physicians in rehabilitative medicine to treat paralysis and muscle weaknesses. In Europe and Canada, these same machines are used not only by physicians but in figure salons for healthy people as an alternative or adjunct to exercise. Carola Barczak has adapted EMS machines for use in the treatment of cellulite by inventing a computer chip that selects and exercises only slow-twitch muscle fibers. Slow-twitch muscle fibers are the long, lean ones found on marathon runners and dancers. They also fuel themselves directly on fat when stressed. A forty-minute session on Barczak's specially designed machines is equivalent to nine hours of exercise. Therefore, fat, which has been made accessible by heat, is used up during the treatments.

This treatment is used on clients with densely packed cellulite. When it has broken up and softened the cellulite, the second treatment (vacusage) follows, as long as the client is at or within ten pounds of her goal weight.

Vacusage encourages lymph drainage and irons and stretches out the underlying warp in the connective tissue so that the fat layer can once again lie flat. Vacusage is widely used in European beauty salons and is now reaching the salons of North America.

In vacusage treatment, vacuum suction is applied externally to the leg. Using a glass suction devise called a *ventouse*, the operator strokes the leg, upward from the knee toward the groin, along the pathways of lymph drainage. She follows a *ventouse* stroke with an upward massage stroke with her free hand. The massage stroke further encourages lymph drainage; it also soothes the discomfort sometimes felt during a client's first few vacusage treatments.

Vacusage treatments should never be applied to legs with enlarged varicose or spider veins. Nor should they be performed on anyone with a history of lymphatic disease. If a vein problem rules out vacusage for you, I recommend first treating the varicose veins with sclerotherapy. Once your varicose veins are taken care of, you may start vacusage. Vacusage should be administered only by skilled professionals—inexperienced application can cause extensive bruising.

Carola Barczak rounds out her treatments with a total-body program. Here is her commonsense regimen for preventing cellulite build-up:

Exercise

A woman with cellulite must choose her exercise routine carefully. Walking and swimming are the best choices because they exercise the slow-twitch muscles and use the whole leg. Jogging also does this, but it makes high demands on the lymph drainage system. Women with a great deal of cellulite more than likely have poor lymph drainage; jogging further taxes an already stressed system.

Bicycling, because it exercises only the quadricep muscles, creates an unbalanced leg, which also stresses lymph circulation. The aerobic exercise portion of an aerobic dance workout is good as long as it continues for more than twenty minutes, which is about how long it takes for your muscles to begin burning fat. Racket sports entail a lot of fast-twitch activity and can aggravate a cellulite problem. Leg weights should be avoided entirely.

Stretching exercises are especially beneficial, as is practicing yoga, which both stretches connective tissue and stimulates lymphatic circulation.

Diet

Cut back on full-fat cheeses and dairy products, marbled beef and pork. (Melted cheese is particularly bad; heat coagulates the protein in cheese, making it less digestible and more constipating.) Eat nuts, seeds, and avocados in moderation.

Eat high-fiber foods. Whole grains, bran, beans, fruits, and vegetables will aid regular elimination. Sluggish bowel function can aggravate a cellulite problem.

Control sodium. Each teaspoon of extra salt in your diet causes your body to retain an extra pound of water. Because of the pull of gravity, most of these fluids will settle in your legs and impair your circulation. Be especially careful about salt in your premenstrual week when the body has a tendency to retain fluids because of high estrogen level.

Cut out sugar. Empty calories from sweets and pastries often result in extra fat and cellulite.

Maintain an adequate protein intake. A low-protein diet will worsen cellulite by causing you to lose muscle and connective tissue and by thinning the walls of lymph and blood vessels. Be sure to include seafood, poultry, eggs, veal, lamb, and liver in your diet. Vegetarians should combine incomplete proteins to ensure adequate protein intake.

Drink six to eight glasses of water a day to maintain fluid balance. Your body loses that fluid each day through perspiration and waste elimination. Also, good lymph drainage depends on adequate water intake.

Drink water between meals rather than with meals. Water taken with food dilutes digestive enzymes and slows digestion. Also, you lose the cleansing effect water has when taken on an empty stomach.

Try to avoid any prescription medications that raise your estrogen level. Birth control pills are the most common source of extra estrogen. Other medications can also aggravate an existing cellulite problem. For instance, chronic use of tranquilizers and muscle relaxants means that your muscles can never really firm up; antihistamines contribute to fluid retention; codeine-based medications are constipating.

Of course, your general health is always more important than getting rid of cellulite, no matter how unattractive it is. Take whatever medications you must for your general good health, but be aware of the effect they may have on your legs.

WHAT YOU CAN'T DO ABOUT CELLULITE

I asked Carola Barczak to evaluate some of the popular products and procedures that claim to remove or reduce cellulite.

She considers the body-wrap a questionable practice. In this process, the body is rubbed down with an "inch-loss" cream and then bandaged in a plastic wrap for one hour. During this hour, body-wrap practitioners maintain, inches and cellulite "disappear." The physiological effect of such treatment is similar to that of bandaging a sprained ankle or wearing a very tight girdle: swelling and fat are compressed and thus temporarily take up less space. But in the following twelve to forty-eight hours—not surprisingly—the body reverts to its pre-body-wrap shape.

She also sees little merit in the widely-advertised cellulite creams, soaps, and scrubbers. These products usually contain extracts of ivy and horsetail, which have a mild diuretic effect on the skin. Diligent scrubbing with the plastic nubby apparatus that holds the extracts may produce some surface smoothing, but too-vigorous scrubbing can result in bruises or spider veins. At best, it is a superficial approach.

The best defense against cellulite is prevention through proper diet, exercise, and habits that keep your lymphatic and venous circulation in good working order. If, however, you have a hereditary tendency toward cellulite or you have acquired it over the years, treatments like Carola Barczak's and vacusage, combined with a regimen of diet and exercise, will help you reduce your current cellulite level and prevent you from developing more cellulite deposits.

13

PIN UP PERFECTION

Liposuction:

plastic

surgery

for

your

legs.

Plastic surgery might not be able to give you pinup-perfect legs, but it can change their contour and thereby enhance the appearance of your legs.

Liposuction, or fat suction, a relatively new plastic surgery technique, removes unwanted pockets of fat that are resistant to exercise and dieting. It can correct "saddlebags" (bulging fat deposits on the sides of your thighs), protruding inner thighs and inner knees, heavy calves, and fatty ankles. Widely used on legs, liposuction can also remove unwanted fat from just about any part of the body.

For the information in this chapter I consulted a fellow physician, Pamela J. Loftus, M.D., a plastic and reconstructive surgeon in Boca Raton, Florida, whose practice centers on cosmetic surgery and liposuction. Dr. Loftus's research on liposuction has earned her an award from the Plastic Surgeon Educational Foundation.

◆ WHAT LIPOSUCTION CAN AND CAN'T DO

First of all, liposuction is NOT a cure for obesity. You cannot arrive at the hospital for liposuction in an obese condition and emerge with legs like Betty Grable's.

Liposuction can and does, however, improve your body contours by removing fat cells. Here is how it works.

As we have learned, the contour of our bodies is largely the result of heredity. Often the shapes of our legs, calves, and hips are patterned after one of our parents.

Similarly, the number of fat cells that are present in our bodies is determined at birth and also, to some extent, by what we eat during childhood. As we grow and develop, the fat cells that we were born with increase in size; as we gain weight our body contour changes accordingly.

Fat cells exist to store excess calories that can be relied on to supply energy for vital body functions. Weight gain and contour deformities are caused by enlargement of the fat cells. Losing weight causes the fat cells to give up some of the liquid oily fluid within them; the fat cells thus shrink in size after weight loss, but they do not disappear or die. As adults, the number of our fat cells tends to stay the same. As our weight goes up or down, only the size of the cells, not the number of them, will increase or decrease. For any permanent change in body contour, therefore, fat cells must be removed.

This is what liposuction does. During the procedure, thousands of fat cells are removed, changing the overall body contour.

◆ WHO SHOULD — AND SHOULDN'T — HAVE LIPOSUCTION

The best results from liposuction are achieved on patients who have good skin tone and elasticity. Motivation is an important consideration: patients with less good skin tone will still be helped by liposuction. Irregularities of the skin will remain in individuals with poor skin tone. However, such women will look better in clothing, but not in a bikini.

Good general health is essential. No one with any serious health problem should undergo liposuction.

◆ HOW LIPOSUCTION IS PERFORMED

Dr. Loftus usually performs liposuction in the hospital, under regional or local anesthesia. If multiple areas are to be suctioned, general anesthesia may be used. The surgeon first outlines with a surgical marking pen the area to be suctioned. Then, tiny incisions, usually less than a half-inch long, are made in the skin. She hides these incisions in a body fold— beneath the buttocks, for instance. Next, she inserts a metal tube through the incision and literally vacuums out fat globules from beneath the skin.

Depending on the amount of fat removed, a patient may go home the same day or Dr. Loftus may have the patient remain in the hospital overnight. Patients with extremely large fatty deposits may sometimes require the operation to be performed in two stages.

◆ AFTER LIPOSUCTION

After liposuction, the patient wears a support garment (an elastic girdle and/or stockings, depending on what areas were suctioned). This garment is then worn for about a month to help the body reabsorb fluid that accumulates beneath the skin after fat suction.

Soreness can be expected around the areas of the suctioning for three to five days. There will be some swelling and bruising of the skin in the area, caused by the movement of the vacuuming tube. Depending on the individual and the extent of the suctioning, swelling and bruising will disappear in the first weeks after surgery.

For a few days after treatment Dr. Loftus recommends that the patient rest, drink fluids, and elevate the legs to promote fluid drainage. A patient can usually resume normal activities in a few days.

The results of liposuction are evident as soon as the support garment is removed and improve visibly as the excess fluid beneath the skin is reabsorbed by the body.

Although many, many fat cells are removed from the suctioned area, some remain. Consequently, if there is a general weight gain, some weight may also be gained in the suctioned area. The area will not, however, return to its pre-liposuction shape. Because there are so many fewer fat cells in that area, it cannot.

◆ IF YOU ARE CONSIDERING LIPOSUCTION

Dr. Loftus emphasizes that fat suction is a safe and excellent procedure when performed by a properly trained plastic surgeon; that is, one who has completed a board-approved residency training of at least two years in plastic and reconstructive surgery.

Some doctors who specialize in other medical fields and are now also performing liposuction have not had the benefit of such extensive residency training in plastic and reconstructive surgery; in fact, some practice liposuction after learning it in a weekend course where they gain no clinical practice in the procedure. This can be very dangerous. To ensure excellent, safe results, make certain the physician you choose to do liposuction has been properly trained.

Fat suction is an advance in plastic surgery that can improve many figure problems.

14

LAST LEGS

Final

encouragement

for

maintaining

your

Great

Legs.

So there you have it: excellent information that, when combined with your common sense and your love and acceptance of your own body, will help you achieve the best legs you can have: *your Great Legs*.

I've stressed the health aspects of leg care in this book because I believe that, first and foremost, Great Legs are healthy legs. You may have been drawn to this book because of a concern with rising hemlines, but let me assure you that using the information in this book will help you maintain your Great Legs long after hemlines have fallen to the floor once more.

Changing your diet and exercise habits will serve you best in the long run, assuming you stick to these new habits. And I'm sure, once you see their effect on your legs (not to mention the rest of you), that you *will* stick to them. You'll get off the junk-food merry-go-round and give your legs the good, wholesome fuel they need to support you and move you ahead in your life. You will exercise regularly, not only for the shape of your legs, but for the overall sense of well-being and satisfaction regular exercise brings.

You can put your best foot forward because you know what to do about a variety of leg concerns. The thought of varicose and spider veins need no longer worry you, because you know how much can now be done to treat them. You also understand the importance of finding and correcting the cause of leg imbalances, which can cause so many secondary problems. You know what causes leg pain and where to go for help when you have it. You have the most up-to-date information about how you get cellulite and what to do about it. And you have the best information available about liposuction, surgical removal of fat.

In the short run, you know how to pamper your legs and yourself with massage and TLC—tender leg care. You can put together a fashion look that will show off your legs to their best advantage.

There is nothing else for me to tell you, except to urge you to use the information in this book. The more you use it, the better the effect on your legs.

Use your common sense, love your legs and yourself, and I am certain you will have excellent results: your Greatest Legs!